THE
MANUAL
HANDLING
REVOLUTION

How health professionals can achieve
creative solutions for people with
disabilities and their caregivers

AIDEEN GALLAGHER

About the author

Aideen Gallagher's vision is to revolutionise the manual handling industry and the process by which allied health professionals recommend manual handling equipment. She is passionate about the mental and physical wellbeing of people with complex physical disabilities and the care workers who assist them.

Aideen is a leader in her field, having published 10 articles in peer-reviewed academic journals. Through her company Risk Managed, she has developed courses in creative equipment prescription and manual handling, called HoistEd and MoveEd, and these are delivered in Australia and Europe.

Aideen is an energetic and engaging presenter. She is recognised for capturing her audience by drawing from her extensive clinical experience and being able to solve the trickiest of problems – and doing so in a way in which everyone wins.

Aideen provides simple insights that are changing the ways thousands of health professionals think about manual handling. Her ambition is that manual handling makes the lives of people with disabilities more comfortable and dignified and the care worker injury free. Aideen's further ambition is that every health professional prescribing manual handling equipment is able to do so with the confidence that they have ensured all parties are safe, while taking every opportunity to eliminate manual handling.

Contact Aideen at aideengallagher@riskmanaged.com.au.

*To Mum and Dad – for making me
believe anything was possible.*

*To my beautiful husband – for supporting
me and making everything possible.*

Acknowledgements

While I always thought I would write a book, I never really believed it would actually happen. No woman is an island and I would not have done this without a massive tribe of people around me to help at various stages of the process. I want to say thank you to all of the following.

Emma Small – for your shared enthusiasm to make the work for caregivers injury free, and for your constant encouragement, ideas and support throughout this whole writing process and beyond.

To all my writing accountability team – Jan Reeves, Dympna Kennedy, Stan Cortes, Mark Ostryn and Rebecca Cribbin – for being with me on those really dark days (and there were loads).

To all at Dent Global – for the mentoring received through the writing process. And to Glen Carlson and Andrew Griffiths – for tricking me into thinking this was going to be easy.

To Kylie Downes and Ann Adams – for giving me the opportunity to work with such an innovative team way back in December 2003 and for teaching me the foundation of what is talked about in this book.

To Emma Small (again!), Clare Webb, Miriam Kolker, Margaret Cullen-Erickson, Todd MacRae, Ellen Cullimore, Helena Travers, Fran Damen and Ann Adams – for taking the time to read my drafts and provide invaluable feedback.

To Guldmann – for the permission to use your diagrams on the front of my book.

To the Canadian Association of Occupational Therapists (CAOT) – for the permission to use the Person–Environment–Occupation–Performance Model to explain my theories

To Charlotte Duff, my editor – for making me feel like this was the most important book you would ever edit. To Peter the designer for your commitment with the cover and Carolyn Bulter Madden for the cover idea. And to Michael Hanrahan and his editing team – for their support beyond just editing and producing this book.

To all the participants of my workshops over the years – for your inspiration and ideas and helping me to increase my knowledge in manual handling. I just love teaching talented professionals.

To all the care workers with whom I have had the pleasure to work during my 15 years as a manual handling advisor – for being the source of most of my knowledge.

And finally to Emile and Luke, my two beautiful boys – for being so patient when I just needed to write and basically surviving on arrowroot biscuits.

First published in 2017 by Aideen Gallagher

Reprinted in May 2018

aideengallagher@riskmanaged.com.au

National Library of Australia Cataloguing-in-Publication entry:

Creator: Gallagher, Aideen, author.
Title: The manual handling revolution.
ISBN: 9781925648263 (paperback)
Subjects: Lifting and carrying – Handbooks, manuals, etc.
           Caregivers – Training of – Australia – Handbooks, manuals, etc.
           People with disabilities – Services for – Australia.
           Older people – Services for – Australia.
           Public health – Handbooks, manuals, etc.

Project management and text design by Michael Hanrahan Publishing
Cover design by Peter Reardon

Disclaimer

The material in this publication is of the nature of general comment only, and does not represent professional advice. It is not intended to provide specific guidance for particular circumstances and it should not be relied on as the basis for any decision to take action or not take action on any matter which it covers. Readers should obtain professional advice where appropriate, before making any such decision. To the maximum extent permitted by law, the author and publisher disclaim all responsibility and liability to any person, arising directly or indirectly from any person taking or not taking action based on the information in this publication.

Contents

PART III: THE TEN PRINCIPLES

Foreword
by Dr Mike Fray

There is an interesting position when an area of scientific investigation develops to such an extent that it supports publications from wider sources. A larger number of publications in books or guidance documents shows a growing level of maturity in the field and is a welcome improvement for all those interested in developing, reviewing or creating their system for managing the risks of moving and handling people in care.

As a researcher and university lecturer my work focuses on the application of ergonomics and human factors in health and community care. For many years it has included work in the development of safe patient handling equipment, methods and systems. This role encourages me to keep informed of the worldwide publications in academic and professional journals and wider publications. To enable the development of our area of interest I am thankful for the addition of this book into this area.

The content and guidance contained is specifically targeted at allied health professionals that are supported by the author's experience and is clearly informed by the author's personal experience. It does specifically engage with the position of therapists in the assessment and prescription of a solution. The structure of the book uses a human-centred approach to the conflicts and challenges of the implementation of safe patient handling. I particularly liked the reference to the emotions that in many ways are barriers to the changes that are required to change how someone is assisted. The management of the expectations of patient, carers, staff, advocates and families can require a significant level of skill and time to allow people the time to change rather than a direct approach of a single assessment and statement of 'this is how it will be'.

One of the specific challenges for rehabilitation professionals is the balance between care handling against delivering or maintaining function. This area is covered in a sensitive way and encourages both carers and patient to consider what is the best outcome in the circumstances. The equipment options we have available currently allow the process to investigate the wider options which may enhance the delivery of a safe, successful and sustainable change in practice. The ten principles in the final section encourage the reader to explore the possible routes to the best solution and should benefit those attempting to implement best practice.

I commend Aideen for her unique approach to the issues around safe patient handling and wish her well on her continued journey to support positive outcomes for all patients, carers, families, staff and organisations involved in the delivery of health and community care.

Introduction

About 12 years ago, I had to assess a client I will never forget. I was working within the Workplace Health and Safety (WHS) department of a care agency as a manual handling advisor. My role was to ensure the agency's care workers were safe when assisting people with disabilities with personal care tasks.

The client I had to assess was 27. He had cerebral palsy and his family was looking for help with his personal care. I noticed straightaway when I looked at the file that this client was born the same day as me. We both started our lives on the same day but, because of his cerebral palsy, his life and the lives of his parents were very different from my life and my parents' lives. How unfair was that.

At the assessment that day, I really wanted to give this family all the help they needed and deserved. However, as part of my role, I had to give the family some news they did not want to hear. The agency was not able to manually lift their son. This resulted in the client's father asking me to leave their home. While I needed to give that message, because of the way I had delivered it I felt I had let them down at a time that they probably needed me most, and I was devastated.

How did this happen, when every bone in my body wanted to make this situation better for this family? I decided that day that I never wanted that to happen again; there must be another way. Manual handling involves moving a person from one position to another, but it is so much more than this. This experience sent me on a path of learning that would change the way I looked at manual handling and how I solved manual handling problems.

Seeing patterns and connections

In the 12 years since that incident, my career has meandered between mental health and manual handling, with a stint in academia along the way. This has allowed me to gain insight into some of the intricacies of the manual handling industry, while also giving me the ability to see the wood from the trees when I stepped out of the industry. I was able to view the situation from an academic perspective when I worked as a lecturer on an undergraduate occupational therapy program, and from a clinical perspective in my various clinical roles. In addition, I have also had the opportunity to work with some really clever professionals, both care workers and health professionals, who have taught me things that have really made a difference to my practice.

Throughout my 15 years in the industry, I have identified certain patterns in the way some allied health professionals address manual handling concerns. These patterns are limiting the extent to which many health professionals can achieve superior outcomes for the client and the care workers who support them, and limiting how confident they feel about the advice they are able to give.

Differing philosophies

I noticed some overarching philosophies in the WHS world that were very different from my practice in mental health. Risk assessment is a process used in both disciplines, yet in mental health it was used more creatively than in manual handling. I studied the literature to see if it was possible to take some lessons from the mental health area and apply them to manual handling. Could we be creative while still having safety as the overarching philosophy?

Focus on people first, then equipment

Allied health professionals I worked with seemed to have the philosophy of using people first and then equipment. I noticed many health professionals were still doing manual transfers when they didn't need to. Equipment was available that completely eliminated the need for manual transfers, and this equipment was easy to use. While many of these resources did cost money, they could be applied to a huge variety of manual handling problems if the clinician was willing to put on their creative hat. The cost of that equipment could eventually be dwarfed by the savings achieved by using the equipment to its fullest potential.

No systematic framework for equipment prescription

Seeing clients in the community with physical disabilities where health professionals were already involved, I started to see patterns in the mistakes some health professionals were making when prescribing equipment. These professionals were lacking a systematic framework, which made mistakes hard to avoid. These mistakes were not resulting in problems with safety, but they were making the carer work harder than they should have had to. In many instances, a second care worker was put in when they were not needed. Watching the way in which the equipment was being used was akin to watching a Ferrari being driven in third gear. With a few minor adjustments to equipment, I knew I would be able to get them up to top gear – with all the benefits for efficiency that had to offer.

I saw that many health professionals weren't confident with equipment. They didn't seem to know what was available and what made one item of equipment different from the other, and what made it most suitable in solving a manual handling problem. Once they had an item of equipment to work with, many didn't know how to make it work for them. While manual handling innovators were coming up with solutions to solve problems, health professionals were becoming overwhelmed with choice.

Increased anxiety

Manual handling was not taught extensively in undergraduate programs, yet health professionals were coming out of university with the expectation that they would be experts in manual handling. Even if a health professional wanted to learn manual handling skills, few postgraduate training options were available to assist them with this upskilling. While improved equipment provided a significant opportunity to eliminate manual handling, no training was available in how to systematically prescribe equipment and ensure the most was made of what it had to offer.

As I started offering manual handling workshops, I noticed an air of anxiety among the health professionals I taught. Many health professionals disliked manual handling and were often fearful about making a wrong decision. Health professionals also felt they were responsible for the actions of a care worker they taught a manual handling routine to – so if a care worker was not following directions, they were to blame.

A manual handling routine aims to control the risk as far as reasonably practicable. The outcome of all risk assessment is that a certain part of the risk remains, no matter what control measures you put in place. Health professionals were becoming anxious about this remaining level of risk when they could not possibly be able to control all the risk, no matter how many skills or resources they had.

Lack of creative thinking

As a lecturer on an undergraduate occupational therapy program, I was aware of the massive emphasis on creative problem-solving in the education of health professionals. Experts in this area recognised this kind of problem-solving was needed for health professionals to be able to adapt to the growing health demands of contemporary practice. While I was confident health professionals had these skills, something appeared to happen when manual handling entered the mix. Some health professionals appeared paralysed and lacked the confidence to apply their demonstrated creative problem-solving skills in a manual handling setting.

Socially and emotionally challenging

As well as being challenging from a physical perspective, manual handling was also socially and emotionally challenging. So many people were involved in the manual handling process – including the client, the care worker and the family. Along with this, the needs for independence and autonomy for the client, and safety for the care worker were sometimes at odds with one another.

In terms of the client, I found that my mental health experience was invaluable to me in my role as a manual handling advisor. This experience gave me the skills to recognise the significant grief many people with disabilities were experiencing when manual handling was involved. Manual handling always involved some kind of loss, where someone was unable to do something they might have been able to do before. I was able to identify this grief and, more importantly, I had the skills to be able to do something about it.

In terms of the care worker, in solving physical problems, I realised very quickly that a manual handling risk can very easily be replaced with a stress risk for the care worker if the way I dealt with the manual handling risk was insensitive towards the client. Care workers were in the client's home and they had to go into that home daily – unlike me, who came in once. I had to ensure my intervention did not add to the stress side of their job through damaging their relationship with their client.

For these reasons, some health professionals were finding manual handling interventions exceptionally challenging. They were the assessments that would take a long time and would involve some kind of conflict. Health professionals would have to manage the needs of multiple parties, without the advantage of some kind of framework for ensuring all needs were met.

The unfortunate result

Allied health professionals were telling me they dreaded the manual handling assessment because they didn't know how to achieve a solution where the client was happy, the care worker was safe and they themselves were confident that they had recommended the best routine possible to meet the needs of all parties.

Health professionals were finding themselves avoiding cases that involved manual handling because they were too challenging and massively complex. Manual handling was the bottom of the barrel in terms of areas to work in.

The manual handling revolution

In 2017, I made the decision to bring all my learning together in a book, and so I present to you 'the manual handling revolution'. This book is the product of my many years of observing, thinking, studying, researching and gaining experience in the care of people with complex disabilities who need a caregiver to move. As an industry, amazing manual handling advisors are out there who really get the big picture. Many gifted therapists come to workshops I run, and they get it and find amazing outcomes for their clients. However, all this is not always filtering down to the general therapist working in the community setting and I wanted to bring to these generalist health professionals a framework for navigating through the maze that is manual handling.

I wrote this book to guide allied health professionals working in the community sector through the process of recommending manual handling routines. My aim is to help these professionals ensure their clients are safe, care workers are resourced and they can leave the office with confidence that they have recommended the best routine they can.

This book explains the client experience of manual handling. It provides a process for meeting client needs with clear signposting so the client can remain in as much control as possible through the process. It discusses the challenges for care workers and why they are at high risk of physical injury and stress. Finally, the book outlines the health professional's experience and how some of their beliefs about manual handling are leading to significant anxiety. *The Manual Handling Revolution* provides a framework for clinicians to address this anxiety, start to be creative and get back to enjoying the job they have to do when assisting people with complex disabilities to move.

The book is divided into three main sections. The first section examines some of the needs of the client, the care worker and health professionals in solving these problems. The second section examines the current risk assessment process used to solve manual handling problems. The final section outlines the ten principles of successful interventions. These principles explain the resources that are at our fingertips and the shift in thinking we need to get to, to be able to get the best out of these resources. Not only will this help reduce injuries, but we will also create efficient and resourceful workers. The principles provide a framework for shifting our thinking to be able to access this process of working. At the end of each principle, I've provided a summary as well as some activities to help you start to implement some of these skills with your team.

10 principles to implement the manual handling revolution

This book explains the ten principles I think are critical to achieving the outcome of a well-resourced care worker, happy client and confident health professional:

1   *Understand it's a negotiation:* Health professionals can feel pulled in different directions, balancing the divergent needs of all parties in the manual handling process. Here I provide a framework for managing this process. This chapter presents the opportunity to create a win–win scenario for the client, family and their caregivers.

2   *Address the grief:* Grief is a significant issue in manual handling, with clients invariably losing something that results in them needing the assistance of a third party. This loss needs to be acknowledged and here I provide a framework for acknowledging this grief, without becoming a formal

counsellor (where this issue takes over the assessment process).

3 *Stop throwing care workers at the problem:* This principle examines the decision to increase care in the home from one care worker to two, and outlines some of the factors we need to consider in making these decisions. While we assume two care workers are better than one, a second care worker introduces many additional complexities that need to be part of the decision-making process.

4 *Manage the manual handling neurosis:* An air of anxiety exists among many health professionals in addressing the manual handling concerns of their clients. In this principle, I provide a framework for managing this anxiety by examining what is in your control and the real aim of risk assessment. I also provide a decision-making framework that compares decisions to the next best alternative to help you examine the best option available and why.

5 *Use systematic assessment:* In getting the best use out of available equipment, I advocate the use of a systematic framework for assessment and for prescribing equipment. Following the same formula for every assessment, you ensure you pick the best product for the problem, taking every opportunity to eliminate manual handling.

6 *Implement objective guidelines:* We need to be able to make objective decisions in the manual handling process, knowing what the client needs to be able to do for the care worker to assist them safely. We need to have a clear guide as to what 'safe' looks like and in turn, what 'unsafe' looks like. This chapter explains how this is as important for the management

of the expectations of parties in the negotiation process as it is for the assessment itself.

7 *Get creative:* In this principle I outline how you can get to intimately know the situation you are assessing. I also outline my framework for creative risk management to start to uncover all the resources and equipment that can help you eliminate manual handling for the care worker and get the best out of the equipment.

8 *Use equipment evaluation to separate the gem from the gimmick:* Here I provide an additional framework to enable clinicians to objectively assess the new manual handling equipment they come across. This framework allows them to take ownership of this assessment without being reliant on others to tell them. This framework forms a model I think we need to start using at conferences to objectively evaluate new equipment that comes on the market.

9 *Consider alternatives to get an outcome:* Manual handling is predominantly a physically orientated discipline and sometimes we think a physical intervention is the only way to solve the problem. This principle is about helping you explore some of the alternative ways to address manual handling concerns without completing any manual handling.

10 *Use the assessment guide:* Finally, I provide a framework for completing an assessment of manual handling need in the home environment. This is to assist you in managing the interests of the client, the family and the care worker, while addressing manual handling concerns in the home.

A note on terms used

Some variation exists in the terms used within the aged and disability section and within manual handling. For clarity, here's how I've used particular terms:

- *Manual handling:* I've used this to capture any task that requires a person to lift, lower, push, pull, carry or otherwise move, hold or restrain any person.[1]

- *Care worker:* While the challenges can be similar for family care givers, in this book I focus mainly on professional caregivers who are paid to provide professional care in the home, and I mostly use 'care worker' when referring to these people. When I use 'caregiver' or 'carer' in the book, I'm referring to the same role.

- *Health professional:* For simplicity, I mostly use 'health professional', 'clinician' or 'therapist' when referring to allied health professionals such as occupational therapists, physiotherapists and workplace health and safety professionals who provide advice on the manual handling of people.

- *Statistics:* This book has been written in the Australian context using statistics from this region. The figures outlined are, in many instances, comparable to those across the developed world.

So now let's get started on the needs of the client, the care worker and health professionals, and how we might look to solve some of the existing problems.

---

1 Workplace Health and Safety (2015). *Hazardous Manual Tasks Code of Practice.* Made under the *Work Health and Safety Act 2011,* section 274. Retrieved 8 August 2017 from www.legislation.gov. au/Details/F2016L00406/Explanatory%20Statement/Text.

Part I

The difficulties with manual handling

This part starts by asking why manual handling is so complicated. I break this question down by looking at all the stakeholders in the manual handling process, discuss the client and their needs, as well as the needs of the care worker and the risks manual handling presents to them. I also outline the changes in the aged and disabilities sectors that are leading to a manual handling 'perfect storm', and conclude by exploring the role of the allied health professional and the expertise expected from them in solving manual handling problems.

Why is manual handling so complicated?

In unpacking the reasons behind manual handling being so complicated, I have found a particular model of practice very useful – although it took me a little while to get there. I was never really a fan of models of practice while at university. I recall writing an essay comparing one model to another and I had no idea what I was writing about. I still didn't know when I left university either. It wasn't until I started working in Aboriginal Health in the Northern Territory of Australia that I really started to understand their application in identifying the source of problems – and, therefore, providing solutions to these problems.

Then, in 2008, I found myself having to teach models of practice to my first-year undergraduate OT students. At first, I was literally one lecture ahead of the students. The more I taught models of practice, however, the more I understood them, and I was determined that no student would leave my class without really getting to understand how a model of practice can help us unpack what might be really going on when we are presented with a mess.

So, how are models of practice connected to manual handling? Since starting my workshops in 2007, I have always received feedback from allied health professionals about how they find manual handling interventions really challenging. These interventions were the ones that were most likely to end up with a complaint and that took so much more time. Most importantly, these situations were the ones therapists most often felt uneasy about – fearing they had let someone down. As a result, many therapists admitted avoiding manual handling cases if possible.

Manual handling interventions are clearly challenging. We all know that and feel it – but why, exactly, are they so hard? I found that the Person–Environment–Occupation–Performance (PEOP) model[1], used to teach occupational therapy practice, explains really well exactly why manual handling is so hard.

The Person–Environment–Occupation–Performance model (the boring stuff)

Before I get stuck into how the PEOP model (outlined in the following figure) relates to manual handling, explaining what is going on in this model is worthwhile. I will refer to this model throughout the book. The model has four main areas or circles, representing the person, their environment, their occupation and their performance. Ideally, they intersect in the middle to create an outcome of health and wellbeing in their occupational performance and participation. Through the arrangement of the circles, the model visually highlights that the person interacts with their environment through the things they do (occupations) and the way they do them (occupational performance) to lead to success or failure (occupational performance and participation).

---

1 Christiansen, CH, Baum, CM & Bass-Haugen, J. (2005). *Occupational therapy: performance, participation, and well-being* (3rd ed). Thorofare, NJ: SLACK.

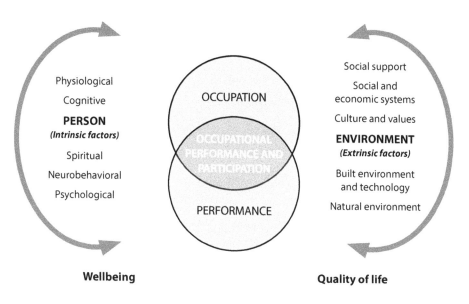

Wellbeing   Quality of life

Reproduced with permission from the Canadian Association of Occupational Therapists (CAOT).

Five main intrinsic elements of a person affect what they bring to this process. (This is not an academic text, so I only explain these areas in basic terms.) The five main areas of personal variables[2] are as follows:

- *Neurobehavioural:* These factors include how we physically move (our motor skills) and what we gain through our five senses (our sensory skills).

- *Physiological:* These involve our endurance, strength and coordination.

- *Psychological and emotion:* These cover our personality traits and our psychological disposition.

- *Spiritual:* What provides meaning to people.

---

2   *ibid.*

- *Cognitive:* These include our levels of attention and the memory aspects that are needed for a task.

The environment in which the occupation occurs brings five main extrinsic elements[3]. These variables are:

- *Built environment and technology:* This area includes buildings and all the physical things in them.

- *Natural environment:* This is the physical world outside the built environment, and the elements of climate that affect it.

- *Culture and values:* This covers cultural ethnicity, factors such as gender, age and socioeconomic background, along with the values that are incorporated into these cultural categories.

- *Social and economic systems:* This includes all public policy aspects and the economic system that has an impact on our lives.

- *Social support:* This covers the emotional and practical support, and the information offered in our environment.

How does this look in manual handling?

If we were to make the PEOP model specific to manual handling, we could say the person interacts with the environment through the manual handling tasks they have to do, and the way they do those tasks ideally leads to a safe and efficient transfer. The figure on the following page outlines what the PEOP looks like when applied directly to manual handling.

While I was teaching this model of practice to my first-year students, one day it came to me that this model could very well explain why manual handling was so hard. I had grown very fond

---

3   *ibid.*

of this model because it was two-dimensional and it was neat. Essentially, one person interacts with their environment through the manual handling routines they do and the way they do them, to lead directly to a safe and efficient transfer.

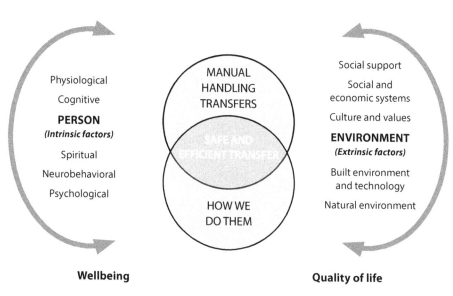

However, manual handling is never a singular activity. The fact that manual handling is needed inherently means that this model completely changes – because someone does not do transfers by themselves. Importantly, *manual handling is always a 'we' activity*, and this makes things a whole lot more complicated. Together, a care worker and their client interact with the environment through the manual handling activities they do, and the way they do them to (ideally) lead to a safe and efficient transfer. A diagram showing this interaction would quickly go from neat to chaos (hence, I have not attempted to do it). The visual chaos in this imagined diagram translates into actual chaos in practice, with the health professional trying to manage all elements of this model – not only for the client but also (and always) for the care worker. In some instances, the situation can involve two care workers and, many times, family as well. As a business leader once told me, once you add an extra person to a process, you haven't just doubled the complexity, but squared it. No wonder the process of manual handling is so hard.

In chapters 2 and 3, I look at each of the two main participants in manual handling (people with disability and care workers) individually, discussing the areas they commonly struggle with.

People with a disability want more

The manual handling PEOP model I outline in chapter 1 (and shown again in the following figure) can describe the situation before a care worker ever gets involved. The client interacts with their environment in the task of moving themselves and how they do this leads to success or failure. If people succeed, they continue as normal. If they fail, allied health professionals get involved, complicating the PEOP model.

In this chapter we highlight how grief and loss can be associated with this failure to be independent. At a time when the barriers to disability are diminishing, we also address the practical implications this change in function has on a person with a disability in their daily activities. Finally, we look at the person of size as a specific group and address some challenges they face if a disability becomes part of their daily life.

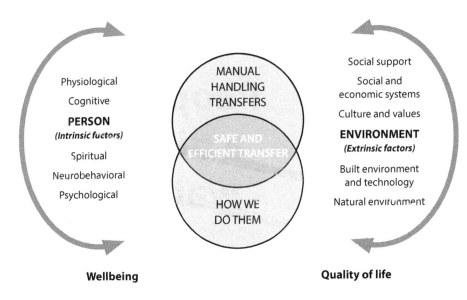

Manual handling can mean moving from ability to disability

As health professionals working in manual handling, we meet a person when they start failing at a fundamental task for them. Often, this task is the ability to move themselves independently, and this failure then influences all the choices that the ability to move independently involves.

Grief and loss

The ability to move yourself is an activity you don't really think about until you lose it. Sometimes this loss happens after an accident; sometimes it happens through a condition that gradually gets worse. But this loss means your movement is now in the hands of another person, so you don't get to have as much choice in when certain activities happen. Sometimes, your care is based on someone else's schedule, with a resultant loss of spontaneity. The greater the loss the person experiences, the greater the assistance they need and the narrower the level of choice the person retains. A significant change occurs, for example, when a person moves from weight-bearing (standing) to non-weight-bearing (non-standing) transfers.

Needing assistance to move is not just about moving or choice, either; it is also about privacy. This movement happens in the context of often the most intimate routines of life – including showering, getting dressed and going to the toilet. The person is now required to invite people, often strangers, into the most intimate parts of their lives. Clients report that at times this can be very confronting.

A manual handling intervention involves some sort of acceptance that independence has not been achieved. In many situations, the client may not be ready to reach this level of acceptance. Sometimes, it is only through the assessments we complete that the person realises that independence may not be achievable and a greater level of external assistance is needed. Other times, they know this themselves but accepting this means addressing how they feel about the impact of their disability on their everyday lives.

Dealing with this loss of personal agency is a grieving process for a person with a disability. This grief can manifest itself in many different ways and, in my work as a manual handling advisor, I have seen a broad spectrum of emotion – from profound verbal outbursts through to complete apathy.

Disability is hard

On top of the grief and loss, living with a disability can be really hard. In Australia, according to the Australian Bureau of Statistics

(ABS), three out of five people with a disability need assistance with at least one activity of living[1]. As well as having implications on how they are moved, and their choice and privacy, an important factor here is also the time they are required to spend on basic activities.

To simply have a shower and get dressed, a person who is not able to stand has to go through the following:

- They have to be rolled to remove their night clothing.

- They have to be rolled to fit a hoist sling.

- They have to be moved in a hoist from their bed into a mobile shower chair.

- They need to be positioned over the toilet.

- They need to be moved into the shower.

- They need assistance with washing.

- They need assistance in drying.

- They have to be moved onto the bed via a hoist after their shower.

- They have to be rolled to get dressed on the bed.

- They have to be rolled to readjust the hoist sling.

- They have to be moved in the hoist off the bed to be transferred into their wheelchair for the day.

If you include activities such as going to the toilet during the day, the total time for personal care can take up to three hours a day.

---

1   Australian Bureau of Statistics (2012). 4430.0 – Disability, Ageing and Carers, Australia: Summary of Findings. Retrieved 2 August 2017 from www.abs.gov.au/ausstats/abs@.nsf/ lookup/3A5561E876CDAC73CA257C210011AB9B?opendocument.

People with disabilities want more

I get the opportunity to work with inspiring people weekly who are doing amazing things in their lives. The lives of people with disabilities are changing. They no longer focus on their disability but rather focus on their ability. Beyond their basic human right to be able to do so, people with disabilities want to achieve and they are succeeding. The physical barriers to disability are also changing. Better access means people with disabilities are able to get to more places. They can get to more workplaces, they can choose more leisure pursuits and they can engage with a larger part of their community.

According to 2015 figures from the Australian Bureau of Statistics (ABS), 53 per cent of people with disabilities aged between 15 and 64 in Australia now participate in the labour market[2]. While people with disabilities have always achieved and participated, the internet age and the advent of social media have broken down many of the remaining barriers to people with disabilities participating meaningfully in life.

Manual handling is the bridge to living

The process of being moved in the morning is the bridge a person with a disability has to cross every single day. They have to endure this transfer process because it is the gateway to them meeting their goals and working on what they want to achieve for the rest of the day.

Alongside this, people with disability also want the freedom from arduous personal care routines, and want to get on with activities that are important to them. Considering personal care is the bridge to achieving goals and aspirations for a person with a

---

2 Australian Bureau of Statistics (2012). *4433.0.55.006 – Disability and Labour Force Participation.* Retrieved 8 August 2017 from www.abs.gov.au/ausstats/abs@.nsf/mf/4433.0.55.006.

disability, we need to make this bridge as short as possible. We also need to ensure this bridge is robust.

People of size also need more

At the time of writing, 63 per cent of Australians are considered overweight or obese[3]. This means that we are seeing a greater proportion of people with a disability who are of size. The combination of disability and size can create added challenges for the manual handling process, especially for the person at the centre of that process.

The loss of function can have significant implications for a person of size, and the inability to weight bear can involve the introduction of equipment. This equipment needs to not only be suitable to the person in terms of their size and their weight, but also fit in and with their environment. For a client I assessed recently, her inability to weight-bear resulted in the home no longer being suitable to meet her needs, because the equipment to support her weight could not fit through the doorways of the home. Of course, not being able to move equipment around the house easily can result in people being confined to their home or even the room in the home in which they sleep.

People of size traditionally have not had a positive experience of the manual handling process, and a number of authors have outlined how people of size can be fearful[4] or unco-operative with the transfer process[5]. Many reports outline people feeling let down by

3   Australian Institute of Health and Welfare (2017). 'Overweight and obesity'. Retrieved 8 August 2017 from www.aihw.gov.au/overweight-and-obesity.

4   Cowley, SP, & Leggett, S. (2010). 'Manual handling risks associated with the care, treatment and transportation of bariatric patients and clients in Australia'. *International Journal of Nursing Practice*, (16), 262–267. doi:10.1111/j.1440-172X.2010.01839.x.

5   Kneafsey, R. (2009). 'The effect of occupational socialization on nurses' patient handling practices'. *Journal of Clinical Nursing*, 9(4), 585–593. doi 10.1046/j.1365-2702.2000.00391.x.

the professionals who are entrusted to care for them. They can even be the brunt of judgemental and discriminatory commentary from health professionals who feel overwhelmed in how to provide them with the care they need[6]. Providing allied health professionals with the resources they need to provide adequate care is a significant step in addressing this judgement and discrimination[7].

In a keynote address at the Australian Association for the Manual Handling of People (AAMHP), Chris Coliviti, a physiotherapist in Queensland Health in Australia, discussed the importance of movement patterns for people of size[8]. Coliviti outlined how people of size move differently from people who are not of size, meaning traditional movement patterns have not been successful in the rehabilitation and subsequent manual handling process for this population. She also discussed the simple omission of the step of 'asking' the person how they normally move and how they think they can assist and be assisted with the transfer process. Sometimes these simple communication strategies are the missing link in the problem-solving process.

The question of hygiene and skin care is of considerable importance to all clients but is even more so for people of size. The pressure on the skin from the increased adipose tissues means the skin is even more vulnerable during the moving process, and the caregiver needs to take extra care that the skin is not compromised as a result. People of size need greater assistance in personal care tasks to adequately clean under and dry skin folds (such as the pannus) because they can be more vulnerable to infection from excessive sweat and fluid leakage through the pores (known as *disaphoresis*).

6   Gallagher, S. (2017). 'Taking the first steps in overcoming bias: Sensitivity, compassion and the obese patient'. Paper presented at the Bariatric Management Innovation Seminar Series, Concord Hospital, Sydney, Australia, 8 February 2017.

7   *ibid.*

8   Coliviti, C, & MacRae, J. (2016). 'Managing Bariatric Patients'. Paper presented at the Australian Association for the Manual Handling of People (AAMHP), Fremantle, Australia, 23 May 2016.

On many occasions that pannus itself can be a similar weight to a limb[9]. As a result of this, allied health professionals and care workers require specific education to be able to manage the needs of this group in an efficient, effective and empathetic manner.

Many equipment options are available to meet the needs of people with disabilities and of size in manual handling. A key component in the process of getting these equipment solutions to where they can be of benefit is the expertise of the health professional sourcing and prescribing them effectively. In chapter 5, I address some of the challenges for allied health professionals in advising on manual handling routines. Another key component of this team is the care worker, and in chapter 3, I discuss some of the difficulties care workers are experiencing while trying to provide quality care to their clients.

---

9   Gallagher, S. (2015). *A Practical Guide to Bariatric Safe Patient Handling and Mobility.* Visioning Publishing.

3

Care workers need more

The process of moving a person with a disability who cannot move themselves always involves the assistance of someone. In many cases, this assistance and care can come from an unpaid person (usually a family member) or from a paid caregiver.

According to 2015 ABS figures, almost 2.7 million Australians are unpaid carers (11.6 per cent of the population). Of those carers, 40 per cent are the partner of the person they are caring for, and 52 per cent are themselves over the age of 65. Taking into consideration parents caring for children and children caring for parents, the average age of the primary caregiver across Australia is 55 years. Over one-third of primary caregivers are living with a disability themselves[1].

The other option is to pay for a carer. While no official statistics for the number of paid caregivers across Australia are available

---

1 Australian Bureau of Statistics. (2016). *3101.0 – Australian Demographic Statistics.* Retrieved 8 August 2017 from www.abs.gov.au/ausstats/abs@.nsf/mf/3101.0.

at the time of writing of this book, the industry is growing. Care workers are usually attracted to this industry because they have a passion for assisting people. They want to give back to their community and make a difference to the life of someone with a disability. Although they can go into the industry with these goals, they can quickly find that they are undervalued, stressed and at high risk of injury.

Caring is physically and mentally hard

The vast majority of tasks in the care of people with physical disabilities involve some kind of manual handling. These activities include bathing, dressing, toileting, feeding, assisted walking and transferring. Within these activities, tasks that involve high exposure to manual handling include repositioning in bed, repositioning in chairs, lifting and holding limbs, and moving equipment[2]. Accounting for all these tasks, performed repeatedly with a number of clients, a significant part of a care worker's day involves some kind of physical assistance. Manually carrying loads of 60 to 100 kilograms is considered high risk in many industries, yet care workers report handling loads of this weight on a weekly basis. And not only are the weights of these loads hazardous, but the unpredictability of a moving load also makes the move even more hazardous. The large exposure to manual handling because of these activities has been consistently linked with the high prevalence of musculoskeletal disorders (MSD) in care workers[3].

The increase in the number of people who are now considered of size also has a significant impact on the physical demands of

---

2   Gallagher, S. (2015). *A Practical Guide to Bariatric Safe Patient Handling and Mobility*. Visioning Publishing.

3   Garg, A, & Owen, B. (1992). 'Reducing back stress in nursing personnel: an ergonomic intervention in a nursing home'. *Ergonomics*, 35(11), 1353–1375. doi: 10.1080/00140139208967398.

even what would have previously been deemed simple activities for care workers. The limb of an obese person can be over 20 per cent of overall weight[4], the same weight as a whole person in some instances. In 1997, Tuhoy-Main calculated that a nurse's typical 8-hour shift involved the cumulative lift in the weight range of 1.8 tonnes[5]. This is likely to be even greater in the current situation, where the proportion of people determined to be of size has steadily increased in the last ten years[6].

As well as caregiving being a physically demanding job, it is also mentally challenging. Much of caring involves dealing with people with intellectual disabilities or cognitive deficits who are very often unable to participate in the practical self-care tasks that the care worker is required to assist with. In many instances, the person with a disability can move against the movements needed for these practical tasks to be completed with ease. Manual handling is as much about the communication of the task as it is about the physical doing of the task. Developing creative ways to positively engage the person with the disability in these practical tasks is a significant mental skill set for a care worker to acquire in reducing the physical demands of caring.

Another aspect to consider is that care workers in the community very often work in the client's own home. While it is the client's home, however, it is also the carer's workplace. Once the care worker walks over the threshold of the door, they are in the client's territory. This can lead to a very subtle shift in the dynamic of power within the home towards the client. When regular care is working

4   Nelson, A, Matz, M, Chen, F, Siddharthan, K, Lloyd, J, & Fragala, F. (2006). 'Development and evaluation of a multifaceted ergonomics program to prevent injuries associated with patient handling tasks'. *International Journal of Nursing Studies*, 43(6), 717–733. doi: 10.1016/j.ijnurstu.2005.09.004

5   Tuohy-Main, K. (1997). 'Why manual handling should be eliminated for resident and career safety'. *Geriaction*, 15, 10–14.

6   Australian Institute of Health and Welfare (2017). 'Overweight and obesity'. Retrieved 8 August 2017 from www.aihw.gov.au/overweight-and-obesity.

smoothly, this may not be of significance and indeed can be quite positive. This power imbalance can pose very real challenges, however, if any conflict, minor or major, arises between the care worker and their client. One factor that can be a source of a conflict, for example, can be a situation where the client's skills deteriorate and a risk to the care worker's health and wellbeing results.

Care workers fill gaps

A person with a disability can be completely dependent on the care worker, who comes into their home to assist them. In providing their personal care, the care worker must achieve the required outcome. They must help the person achieve a safe and comfortable position before they leave, whether that is in bed or in their chair. The person can't be 'half positioned'. No matter how difficult getting to that outcome is, unless the risk of injury is immediately obvious where they can say no, care workers don't have a choice – they need to get that outcome.

As illustrated in the following figure, when a client and care worker interact in a personal care task, both bring skills to the process. This interaction allows the care worker to assist the client in reaching the outcome of a safe and efficient transfer. Challenges occur, however, if the client's condition deteriorates. When the client is unable to contribute like before, a gap ultimately occurs that results in a failure of the transfer. The situation then evolves where the care worker starts to fill the gap created by the deterioration in the client's condition. Sometimes the amount of assistance they are providing to fill this gap is masked. You can't necessarily push equipment beyond what it is capable of doing, but you can push a person.

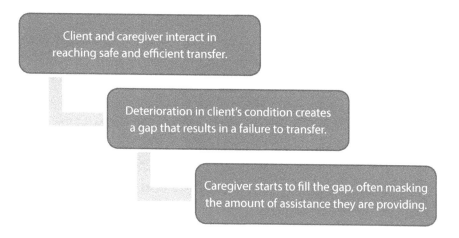

Client and caregiver interact in reaching safe and efficient transfer.

Deterioration in client's condition creates a gap that results in a failure to transfer.

Caregiver starts to fill the gap, often masking the amount of assistance they are providing.

Care workers can find themselves at significant risk of injury by compensating for the skills the client is losing to allow the transfer to continue as previously.

The limitations of the hazard report form

Care workers are versed in the procedures of reporting on the kind of situation outlined in the previous section. Standard practice involves the submission of a hazard report form to management, reporting the source of the problem and a suggestion on what to do about it.

Historically, health agencies have faced significant challenges in the submission of the hazard report form[7]. In the manual handling training I regularly provide, for example, some care workers tell me they are very unlikely to submit a hazard report form in a situation such as this because they don't want to be seen to be complaining or informing on the client when their function has deteriorated. They feel the client could misinterpret the reporting as an attack on themselves, their skills or their home. They know the hazard report

---

7   Collins, M. (1990). 'A comprehensive approach to preventing occupational back pain among nurses'. *Journal of Occupational Health and Safety Australia and NZ*, 6(5), 361–368.

form will solve the manual handling risk, but the client being forced to change the way they do things is likely to replace this risk with a new stress risk. Care workers can find themselves at times blamed for this change.

Care workers can form a significant relationship with the client they provide care for. It can be an overwhelmingly stressful job and when a care worker forms a positive relationship with a client, they don't want to jeopardise that. Many care workers I have talked to describe submitting a hazard report form and, as a result, damaging what was a strong, trusting relationship with their client. Often, they say, this relationship never recovers.

Injuries among care workers

We know a correlation exists between increased exposure to manual handling tasks and musculoskeletal disorders (MSD)[8]. This means the more complex the manual handling we ask care workers to do, the greater the chance they will be injured. Manual handling injuries already account for 29 per cent of all workplace injuries in New South Wales. Health and social care workers have the highest number of workplace injuries, with over 3,500 in 2012–13. In this sector, manual handling injuries cost $104 million per year in New South Wales and result in 68,798 weeks of lost productivity[9]. A 2007 Canadian study found that care aides were at greater risk of injury than nurses, with 37 injuries per 100 full-time staff[10]. Further research has shown that possible reasons for this greater risk

---

8   Marras, W, Davies, K, Kirking, B. & Bertsche, P. (1999). 'A comprehensive analysis of low back disorder risk and spinal loading during the transferring and repositioning of patients using different techniques'. *Ergonomics*, 42 (7), 904–926.

9   Workcover (2012/13). 'Statistical bulletin 2012/13 – NSW workers compensation statistics'. Retrieved 8 August 2017 from www.opengov.nsw.gov.au/publications/14319.

10 Alamgair, H, Cvitovich, Y & Yassi, A. (2007). 'Work related injury among direct care occupations in British Columbia, Canada'. *Occupational and Environmental Medicine*, 64 (11), 769–775. doi: 10.1136/oem.2006.031914

include less training, lower status, and less control or support in their workplace[11].

In addition, anxiety and stress disorder were the highest occupational diseases in the general population that lead to absence from work in 2012–2013 in New South Wales. Within this figure, care workers reported the second highest prevalence of anxiety and stress disorder by occupational group. So care workers are at risk of not only physical injury, but also mental distress. These two factors combined make this group in the Australian workforce one that is dealing with significant risk of injury.

Musculoskeletal injury can have a tremendous impact on the life of a care worker – physically, psychologically and socially. It can result in temporary or permanent physical disability that can involve significant chronic pain. This can result in prolonged sickness or the inability to continue in the caregiving role, leading to job loss and psychological problems such as depression. This can not only affect the carer's work life, but also influence their personal life, resulting in the inability to complete the important activities of daily living. Recognising the economic and social cost of injuries, and the anxiety and stress it involves, prevention is critical in managing this workplace health and safety concern. Care workers have the right to go home to their families, injury free.

---

11 Pompeii, LA, Lipscomb, HJ, Schoenfisch, AL, Dement, JM. (2009). 'Musculoskeletal injuries resulting from patient handling tasks among hospital workers'. *American Journal of Industrial Medicine*, 52(7), 571–578. doi: 10.1002/ajim.20704.

4

The manual handling perfect storm

In the coming years, aged and disability services will face a significant challenge. They will need to supply a high standard of care to people, on a limited budget with reduced staff resources. This comes at a time when the number of people requiring that care will increase and their care needs will become more complex. We are aspiring to do all this within the community sector with a focus on 'the home'.

Aged care and disability is changing

In aged care, we have shifted our focus to a policy of 'ageing in place'[1]. Older people want to live in a familiar environment, usually the traditional family home, and want to avoid residential

---

1   Heumann, LF, & Boldy, DP. (1993). 'The basic benefits and limitations of an aging-in-place policy'. In Heumann LF, Boldy DP, eds. *Aging in Place with Dignity: International Solutions to the Low-Income and Frail Elderly.* London: Praeger, 1–8.

aged care[2]. Similarly, the disability sector is seeing a push towards community care. The National Disability Insurance Scheme (NDIS) in Australia, for example, promotes a participant-centred scheme, enabling people to live in the community with the supports needed to make this happen. It allows the person with a disability to manage their own funding and choose what providers assist them. The NDIS recognises that people with disabilities just want to be able to live an ordinary life. According to Professor Rhonda Galbally, 'there are things everyone takes for granted, and it is those things that are ordinary that ought to be ordinary for people with disability too'[3].

Increased demand on services

Health spending now represents a greater proportion of the Australian economy than ever before[4]. In 2014–15, $161.6 billion was spent on health goods and services; in the same year, health spending reached 10 per cent of Australia's gross domestic product (GDP) for the first time. Home care in the community is a component of this spend and includes the aged and disability sector.

There were around 3.5 million older Australians in 2015, representing one in every seven people or 15.1 per cent of the population[5]. From 1946 onwards, Australia (like most of the Western world) experienced a baby boom, with more than 4 million Australians born between 1946 and 1965[6]. In 2016, the first of these baby boomers started turning 70, and 53 per cent of older Australians

---

2   Hansen, E.B. & Gottschalk, G. (2006). 'What makes older people consider moving house and what makes them move?' *Housing, Theory and Society*, 23(1), 34–54.

3   National Disability Insurance Agency (2016). 'Towards an ordinary life'. Annual Report 2015–16. Retrieved 8 August 2017 from www.ndis.gov.au/medias/documents/ha5/h04/8798853726238/ NDI7040-AnnualReport2016-vFaccessible.pdfpage 2.

4   Australia Institute of Health and Welfare (2017). 'Latest health spending figures reveal mixed trends'. Retrieved 8 August 2017 from www.aihw.gov.au/media-release-detail/?id=60129557213.

5   Australian Bureau of Statistics (2016). *3101.0 – Australian Demographic Statistics*. Retrieved 8 August 2017 from www.abs.gov.au/ausstats/abs@.nsf/mf/3101.0.

6   *ibid.*

reported a disability[7]. With a correlation between age and disability, the number needing care is expected to continue to rise for the next 25 years.

Home care services are also expected to rise. According to the Federal Government's Australian Institute for Health and Welfare, the number of people accessing home care in the aged sector rose by 43 per cent between 2010 and 2015 (from 50,800 to 72,700). This in turn has resulted in increased investment in the sector, with government spending on aged care increasing by 44 per cent between 2009–10 and 2014–2015. In 2014–15, home support services and home care accounted for a combined spend of $3.2 billion[8]. And Australia is going to continue investing in home-based models of care as the number of people with disabilities increase.

Australia already has 4.3 million people living with a disability, and three out of five Australians need assistance with at least one activity of daily living. According to the ABS, almost one-third of these people have a profound or severe disability[9]. As mentioned, the introduction of the NDIS means that, into the future, the vast majority of these people will live in the community. As of 30 June 2016, from the trial and early transition NDIS sites, 35,695 participants were registered with NDIS. The average annual participant package cost was $36,049. When the NDIS is fully implemented in 2019, $22 billion will be spent per year supporting around 460,000 participants with a disability[10].

As mentioned in chapter 2, 63 per cent of Australians are classified as overweight or obese. Along with ageing Australians, obesity

7   Australian Institute of Health and Welfare (2017). 'Ageing'. Retrieved 8 August 2017 from http://www.aihw.gov.au/ageing.

8   Australian Institute of Health and Welfare (2017). 'Aged care spending'. Retrieved 8 August 2017 from www.aihw.gov.au/aged-care/residential-and-home-care-2014-15/aged-care-spending.

9   Australian Bureau of Statistics (2015). 4430.0 – Disability, Ageing and Carers, Australia: Summary of Findings. Retrieved 8 August 2017 from www.abs.gov.au/ausstats/abs@.nsf/mf/4430.0.

10 National Disability Insurance Agency (NDIS, 2016). op cit.

appears to be another upward trend – moving from 56.3 per cent of Australians in 1995 to 61.2 per cent in 2007–08. Of people aged between 65 and 74 years, 74.95 per cent report being overweight or obese. It is not only adults who are experiencing obesity, however; 25 per cent of Australian children are considered to be in the overweight or obese range[11]. Significant challenges present themselves when disability and obesity mix. And, according to Muir and Archer, the increased demands of people of size on our health system lead to an increased need for time, skill, workers and equipment[12].

Future demands on the aged and disability sectors

We are entering a manual handling perfect storm because:

1   The push for care in the community in both aged and disability sectors means we are going to need more care workers than ever before to meet this increased demand as the population ages.

2   We are getting more obese, resulting in increased complexities in the care we need to provide.

3   We are being warned of an imminent crisis in the aged and disability sector, caused by a lack of care workers to meet this demand.

These sectors have struggled to attract and retain workers due to the relatively low pay rates and lack of secure employment

---

11 Australian Institute of Health and Welfare (2017). 'Overweight and obesity'. Retrieved 8 August 2017 from www.aihw.gov.au/overweight-and-obesity.

12 Muir, M, & Archer-Heese, G. (2009). 'Essentials of a bariatric patient handling program'. *Online Journal of Issues in Nursing*, 14(1), 1. doi: 10.3912/OJIN.Vol14No1Man05.

opportunities[13]. As discussed in chapter 3, the high prevalence of injury makes this sector even more unattractive.

The benefits of care in the community for people with disabilities and the aged care population occur at an individual and a community level, both economically and socially. We therefore need to have adequate staff resources to meet the increasing demand. If we are to recruit and retain care workers in these roles, we also need to get over the added barrier of high rates of physical injury coupled with rates of psychological distress.

The opportunity

The research base in manual handling is comprehensive, and a large body of evidence shows that safe patient handling programs are effective in reducing injuries in manual handling[14, 15, 16]. Assistive technology is a critical part of the effectiveness of these programs[17] and allied health professionals are entrusted with the role of identifying the needs for this equipment, prescribing the most appropriate item and training carers on the most efficient and effective use of this item.

13 Harrington, M, & Jolly, R. (no date). 'The Crisis in the caring workforce'. Retrieved 8 August 2017 from www.aph.gov.au/About_Parliament/Parliamentary_Departments/Parliamentary_Library/pubs/BriefingBook44p/CaringWorkforce.

14 Nelson, A, Matz, M, Chen, F, Siddharthan, Lloyd, J & Fragala, G. (2005). 'Development and evaluation of a multifaceted ergonomics program to prevent injuries associated with patient handling tasks'. *International Journal of Nursing Studies*, 43(6), 717–733. DOI:10.1016/j.ijnurstu.2005.09.004.

15 Theis, JL, & Finkelstein, MJ. (2014). 'Long term effects of safe patient handling program on staff injuries'. *Rehabilitation Nursing*, 39(1), 26–35. doi: 10.1002/rnj.108.

16 Garg, A, and Owen, B. (1992). 'Reducing back stress in nursing personnel: an ergonomic intervention in a nursing home'. *Ergonomics* 35(11), 1353–1375. DOI: 10.1080/00140139208967398.

17 Chhokar, R, Engst, C, Miller, A, Robinson, D, Tate, RB, Yassi, A. (2005). 'The three year economic benefits of a ceiling lift intervention aimed to reduce healthcare worker injuries'. *Applied Ergonomics*, 36(2) 223–9. DOI:10.1016/j.apergo.2004.10.008.

The skill set of these professionals is critical to the effectiveness of safe patient handling programs – that is, in getting the right resources, with the right information to the care worker/client team who needs it. In chapter 5, I outline some of the challenges facing health professionals fulfilling the role of experts in addressing complex manual handling problems.

Where are we as allied health professionals in all of this?

In the previous chapters, I outlined the impact of manual handling on people with disabilities and their caregivers, and how allied health professionals are facing an oncoming 'perfect storm' in future manual handing needs. So how are health professionals feeling as they face this future? Many tell me they feel anxious about addressing manual handling concerns with their clients. They report feeling like they don't have the skills to deal with manual handling issues, even though they are considered the expert on the health team in manual handling. They feel the job is getting more challenging with the moving and handling problems they are facing. They find balancing the needs of both parties – that is, care workers and people with disabilities – really difficult. They find manual handling cases are most likely to be the really drawn-out cases, leading to 'assessment creep' and taking up much of their emotional and physical energy. I think if we recognise the roots of the issues, we can then determine what we can do about them.

Manual handling is considered a science, with many guide-lines or hard facts contributing to our knowledge. I think there is another side to manual handling and this is the art. These are the set of softer skills needed to navigate our way through problems. In this chapter, first we will look at some of the science-based factors for health professionals in addressing manual handling problems.

Third-level education

The reality is that health professionals (such as occupational thera-pists and physiotherapists) are considered experts in manual han-dling when they leave university[1]. However, while manual handling is a major skill set for health professionals, very little training on it occurs in university. When I was lecturing in an undergraduate pro-gram, students were offered one day of manual handling training. The curriculum still doesn't have room for everything the health professional needs to know. Even if it did have room, as Moulton suggests, the university structure is a conveyer belt of skills marked by massed practice, where students learn a massive number of skills with an even greater gap between the time when they learn the skill and when they use it[2].

Education is, however, a lifelong journey of learning, as opposed to something that starts and ends at university[3]. The Australian Health Professional Registration Agency (AHPRA) estab-lished registration for occupational therapists and physiotherapists in 2012, and this move to registration can be seen worldwide. This

1   Darragh, AR, Campo, M, & Olson, D. (2009). 'Therapy practice within a minimal lift environment: perceptions of therapy staff'. *Work*. 33(3), 241–53. doi: 10.3233/WOR-2009-0872.
2   Moulton, C, Dubrowski, A, MacRae, H, Graham, B, Grober, E, & Reznick, R. (2006). 'Teaching Surgical Skills: What Kind of Practice Makes Perfect?' *Annals of Surgery*, 244 (3):400–409. doi: 10.1097/01.sla.0000234808.85789.6a.
3   Fletcher, SW. (2008). Chairman's summary of the conference. 'Continuing education in the health professions: improving healthcare through lifelong learning'. *Journal of Continuing Education in Nursing*. 39(3):112–8.

step acknowledges two things. Firstly, our need as allied health professionals to keep abreast of research advances in our field so we can ensure we are giving the best possible care to our clients. Secondly, that we don't know everything and some skill sets are learnt after graduation. The continued education required through registration is important not only because knowledge can change, but also because if we are not using the skills we have learnt, we eventually lose them.

Increased complexity

As noted in earlier chapters, many more people with disabilities are living actively in the community compared to the past[4]. We have to provide a high level of quality care, sometimes with limited resources and in environments that are not specifically designed for this purpose.

Some allied health professionals report feeling overwhelmed at the sheer scale of the challenges they are now required to address; for example, the client of size. As mentioned in chapter 2, studies have shown that judgement and discrimination of people of size are prominent in health services[5]. Staff attitudes and judgements improve significantly, however, when they feel supported and resourced to deal with the problems. According to Susan Gallagher (no relation), expert in the safe moving and handling of the client of size, these supports and resources come in the form of equipment and procedures. As noted by Gallagher, we have all the equipment resources we need to address these manual handling concerns – we are just not using them[6].

---

4   Milner, P, & Kelly, B. (2009). 'Community participation and inclusion: People with disabilities defining their place'. *Disability and Society*, 24(1), 47–62. doi: 10.1080/09687590802535410.

5   Gallagher, S. (2017). 'Taking the first steps in overcoming bias: Sensitivity, compassion and the obese patient'. Paper presented at the Bariatric Management Innovation Seminar Series, Concord Hospital, Sydney, Australia, 8 February 2017.

6   Gallagher, S. (2017). 'The needs of the person living with obesity'. *op cit.*

Two very different needs

As allied health professionals, our involvement with a person with a disability in the activity of manual handling can place us in two camps. Firstly, our role can be for the person, where we are working with the client to support their goals in the manual handling process. Secondly, we can also find ourselves working for the care worker, like I was, from the workplace health and safety (WHS) perspective. Initially, the needs of both can appear to be at odds with one another, and health professionals report feeling confused about their role in manual handling situations.

In my 15 years in the industry, I have seen some masters in the manual handling field achieving excellent outcomes for their clients. I have also seen first hand that sometimes health professionals simply don't know what they don't know.

In allied health professions, the goal of treatment is essentially to rehabilitate and promote independence[7]. In the rehabilitation role, the health professional takes on the role of interim care worker in supporting rehabilitation. This can mean challenging patients to stretch beyond their capabilities with an aim to restore function or maintain it. Manual handling can seem contradictory to this goal because it is doing the opposite – it is taking away someone's freedom to move themselves the way they want to be moved.

A 2009 study found health professionals see equipment as a step backwards in rehabilitation and the aim is to wean patients off equipment as soon as possible[8]. This means the care worker replaces equipment. This is in an age when we have seen massive advances in overhead hoist systems installable in almost any environment

---

7 Radomski, MV, & Trombly Latham, CA. (2008). *Occupational Therapy for Physical Dysfunction*. Wolters Kluwer. Lippincott Williams & Wilkins.

8 Darragh, AR, Huddleston, W, & King, P. (2009). 'Work-Related Musculoskeletal Injuries and Disorders among Occupational and Physical Therapists'. *The American Journal of Occupational Therapy*, Vol 63 (3), 351–362.

(my colleague has just installed one in a shed). These systems can support independent walking, self-transfers, graded exercises and rolling, eliminating the need for the health professional to place themselves at risk. The study found that transfers supported by a health professional, however, are seen as more patient focused and true to their professional philosophy of promoting independence[9].

This study also found an inherent belief among allied health professionals that good body mechanics alone meant it was possible to safely perform certain lifting tasks. Many studies have shown this isn't the case[10] and that therapists have inadequate knowledge and skills in injury prevention[11]. This misguided belief results in health professionals taking considerable risks when working with their patients, especially given the prevailing view among allied health professionals that the patient comes first.

Therapists still consider the patient to be their prime focus, as opposed to self-care and maintenance of health. A 2002 study also found that when an allied health professional gets an injury, they are unlikely to tell their manager or take any time off work[12]. What they are likely to do is blame themselves for the injury and their lack of good body mechanics[13]. They are also likely to try to self-manage the injury themselves, as opposed to going for professional help[14].

---

9 ibid.

10 Marras, WS, Davis, KG, Kirking, BC, & Bertsche, PK. (1999). 'A comprehensive analysis of low-back disorder risk and spinal loading during the transferring and repositioning of patients using different techniques'. *Ergonomics*, 42(7), 904–926.

11 Australian Physiotherapy Association (2003). 'APA Position Statement: Prevention of work related conditions in physiotherapists'. Camberwell, VIC: APA.

12 Passier, L, & McPhail, S. (2011). 'Work related musculoskeletal disorders amongst therapists in physically demanding roles: qualitative analysis of risk factors and strategies for prevention'. *BMCbMusculoskeletal Disorders*, 25(1); 12:24. doi: 10.1186/1471-2474-12-24.

13 Cromie, JE, Robertson, VJ, & Best, MO. (2002). 'Work-related musculoskeletal disorders and the culture of physical therapy'. *Physical Therapy*, 82(5), 459–472.

14 Passier, L, & McPhail, S. (2011). *op cit.*

When is care rehabilitation and when is it functional transfers?

I have been asked to assess a transfer regime on many occasions when a rehabilitation team has recommended a two-person sit-to-stand transfer with a pelican belt. This can be for a client who is inconsistently weight bearing, meaning the care workers are often required to take the client's weight to transfer them into standing. Some clients can consistently help with the transfer and some cannot.

When making decisions in situations like this, the reasoning is that if the client does not weight bear, they will lose their ability to do so. Standing transfers are, therefore, advised where the care worker assists – with the aim that carers are helping to maintain function by allowing the client a certain level of standing tolerance a day. Considering that standing transfers can be a maximum of ten seconds, it is questionable whether 60 seconds of standing tolerance a day (at most) reaches the threshold for meaningful rehabilitation. Of course, this can also be coupled with walking practice with two care workers each side. However, if the person is not able to consistently weight bear in the first place, this practice significantly increases the risk of falls and subsequent injury for all parties. We then enter a vicious circle where the client is not getting enough standing tolerance for walking to improve, and so the risk of injury when they are getting this exposure to walking stays at a high level or continues to deteriorate further. A specific rehabilitation program that addresses deficits in function in addition to functional transfers is missing. In other words, functional transfers are seen as the rehabilitation.

Safe manual handling is contradictory to this philosophy, because it involves taking away the freedom someone has to be independent in tasks involving moving themselves. This concept itself is really at odds with everything that allied health profession-als learn in terms of their goals with clients, and this dissonance can be a challenge to work through conceptually.

'Safety' is something that is regularly mentioned in manual han-dling but, often, without a definition of what safety actually means. The line between 'safe' and 'unsafe' can depend on the opinion of the health professional making that call. Because safety can be a reason to take away something from the client, the client can feel their rights have been infringed based only on a subjective decision made by the health professional. With misinformation sometimes guiding these decisions, recommendations can appear contradictory to the client – for example, when two different professionals have two very different opinions. This can lead to a misinterpretation where a therapist is seen as being 'for' or 'against' rehabilitation, leading to a contradiction for health professionals and their sense of their role. This can fracture a therapeutic relationship, at a time when it is needed the most.

Equipment

We now have the most amazing equipment at our fingertips, which can help to eliminate the need for us or care workers to use their bodies to assist someone. Equipment solutions have been found to be effective at reducing exposure to manual handling[15]. Although these resources are there, we have two problems. Firstly we don't always have the basic knowledge by which to use the equipment and so the confidence in using it with clients. Secondly, we don't have the confidence by which to keep extending that knowledge and start to work with the equipment to challenge how much it can actually do for us.

---

15 Chhokar, R, Engst, C, Miller, A, Robinson, D, Tate, RB, Yassi, A. (2005). 'The three year economic benefits of a ceiling lift intervention aimed to reduce healthcare worker injuries'. *Applied Ergonomics*. 36(2), 223–229. DOI: 10.1016/j.apergo.2004.10.008.

Although equipment has the potential to solve problems, it is costly if prescribed incorrectly or used inefficiently, meaning unnecessary manual handling still exists. What is considered safe on paper can be unsafe in practice where simple opportunities to avoid manual handling are missed. This can lead to a greater number of care workers than would otherwise be required, leading to unnecessary costs with staff resources that are in short supply. As health professionals, we need to be able to prescribe equipment effectively and make it attractive for the care workers using it. Sometimes the safety benefits are not enough; we need to be able to promote efficiency. In other words, we need to show how the bridge to living for the client can be made as short as possible, and how the process can create a safe and efficient working environment for the care worker.

Policies and guidelines

Policies and guidelines have sought to offer some direction in terms of how a person with a disability should be moved. The manual handling industry itself has experienced a number of conversations in prioritising the rights of each party (carer and person with disability). Before the 1980s, standard practice would have been the carer lifting and supporting the person with the disability in activities. Equipment was quite poor at the time so people would fill the gaps for the person with the disability. With the mounting manual-handling-related injuries causing permanent disablement for the person giving care, the balance tipped towards the care worker.

The advent of the 'no lift' policy resulted in a push for no lifting of any patient, and this soon became blanket policy across health services. The aim was to replace manual lifting with the use of a mechanical aid. However, people experienced many adverse effects because of this blanket policy; for example, reports of people not being lifted when they needed to be were widespread in the media at the time.

The policy then changed again to a 'minimal lift' policy. While this policy still did not advocate for lifting, it did suggest an assessment would need to take place first to determine if there could be justification for lifting – that is, where a mechanical aid did not do the job.

Discussions and guidelines in manual handling for how a person should be moved have also addressed the decision to mobilise a person who is unable to weight bear. Decisions whether it was safe to mobilise a client or not were previously made based on the health and safety risk posed to staff. However, as Cohen and colleagues point out in their white paper on assessment of moving and handling, the cessation of mobilisation can result in a greater health and safety risk for staff due to the added dependency it creates – ultimately requiring increased manual handling. This is resulting in a push-back towards facilitation of mobilisation and the use of assistive devices – as opposed to the assistance of care workers – to reach this aim[16].

We have great equipment solutions for those mid-tier transfers that require partial weight bearing. This equipment includes items such as standing hoists and standing pivot aids. Although we have some great resources, still very few guidelines exist for allied health professionals on when an item of equipment is safe for both a care worker and the person they are assisting. Assessment for some of these devices can sometimes neglect to account for hazardous transfers, such as a lying to sitting transfer, that are an essential requirement for some of these sit to stand transfer aids to be functional.

---

16 Cohen, MH, Nelson, GG, Green, DA, Leib, R, Matz, MW, Thomas, PA et al. (2010). 'Patient Handling and Movement Assessments: A White Paper'. Faculty Guidelines Institute. Retrieved 8 August 2017 from www.fgiguidelines.org/wp-content/uploads/2015/08/FGI_PHAMA_ whitepaper_042810.pdf.

* * *

Many of the challenges we have discussed so far could be considered the scientific side of manual handling. Now let's look at those considered the artistic or softer skills of manual handling.

Elephant in the room – we are in the business of giving bad news

After my experience with the 27-year-old client discussed in the introduction to this book, I realised in my role as a manual handling advisor that I was in the business of giving people bad news. It involved taking away the right to stand and the right to set goals that involved working towards independence. The key thing to remember here is that manual handling involves loss. People are losing something and we are the ones as health professionals who have to give that bad news. From the workshops I run, some therapists tell me they feel at sea during this process. They feel someone is going to have to lose, whether that be the client or the care worker. With WHS advocating for the care worker, the person to lose is more often than not the client.

However, this situation gives us the greatest opportunity to walk with someone at a time when they most need our support. The facts of someone's situation don't change, no matter how much we want them to. In many instances, they have reached a stage where they will not be able to participate in a transfer routine the way they were. We are just the first person to call it. Disability is hard and we need a way of showing our respect, sensitivity and compassion while empowering the client where we can through the process.

Working with staff and carers

As allied health professionals, we are assisting carers who are working in very challenging circumstances. As previously discussed, many care workers will have chosen to take on the carer role because they want to give back and offer something to society. Unfortunately, they can quickly learn they have entered a career that is undervalued and with a high incidence of injury as well as psychological stress. As health professionals providing support to the clients or the care workers themselves, we are sometimes bombarded with challenges that emerge when implementing interventions that can, on paper, look quite straightforward.

I was asked to intervene in a case where a health professional was trying to change a weight-bearing client's equipment from a bath shower trolley, which had been used by staff for years, to a shower chair. The argument was that showering while sitting was more dignified for the client, because they had the ability to sit independently as well as transfer onto and off a chair almost independently. However, this intervention caused massive resistance from staff. The health professionals were completely perplexed as to why the staff might react this way.

The staff and carers who work with people who are physically and mentally disabled do a fantastic job. It is an exceptionally challenging role that can be both physically and mentally exhausting. Sometimes carers are so overwhelmed with what they have to do that they don't want anything to change. Whatever they have to deal with in their present, no matter how challenging it is, it is a known quantity. They know the challenge and, since they are doing it, they are comfortable that they can manage it. They resist any change because they do not always feel confident this change will *not* make things harder.

As health professionals, we recommend and then discharge. The staff and carers don't. They have to provide care today and tomorrow in the same way they did yesterday. Care workers have at times described feeling abandoned by health professionals who make recommendations based on one-off assessments and make changes to routines that look great on paper but are a disaster in practice. A new solution making the care worker's role more difficult than it was before can be exceptionally challenging to a staff member who is already completely overwhelmed with what they have to do.

Another aspect is at play in these scenarios. Many care workers form significant therapeutic relationships with their clients and they would do anything for them – sometimes beyond what is safe and to the detriment of themselves. Replacement of their care with an equipment solution can be a challenge for this care worker, even though from a WHS perspective it is mandated.

Introducing change in these environments involves a lot of listening to the care worker and tuning into their concerns, to understand the 'whys' and the 'why nots' in terms of care worker behaviour when assisting with certain tasks. We need to gain their trust, and then respect that trusting relationship when it is given to us. We need to educate collaboratively to enable them to make positive and sustainable decisions towards safety in their everyday work.

Assessment creep

Given the various components of the allied health professional's role in manual handling, many participants of my courses report manual handling–specific referrals can be the most complex ones.

While they look relatively straightforward on paper, the assessments often take longer than expected while managing the needs of everyone. They can be more stressful and can regularly end up with some kind of conflict. This can lead to 'assessment creep' – a term coined by an occupational therapy colleague – meaning that a case trickles along well after the original assessment has taken place and engulfs a massive amount of the therapist's time. Often, the therapist cannot really figure out why it is so intense and what they can do about it.

Dealing with 'assessment creep' demands a strategy where the physical as well as the social and emotional elements of the assessment process are managed. This involves planning to take control of these elements to achieve not only an effective intervention, but also an efficient and timely one.

Dealing with anxiety

Risk assessment is the process we use to solve manual handling problems. The problem we are trying to solve is the risk of injury to the carer. This involves determining a transfer routine for the client and their carer that is safe, yet one that does not impinge on the right of the client to independence. The very nature of manual handling involves dealing with risk and the assessment of risk. A lot of fear can exist among allied health professionals about assessment outcomes where risk still remains.

A number of health professionals who attend my courses report lying awake at night worrying about the risk that remains after doing an assessment. They fear the call reporting that a care worker sustained an injury because of the independence that a client was assessed to maintain. They also fear a complaint from the client whose rights in the assessment process were felt to be infringed so as to protect the health and wellbeing of the care worker. Either way, many allied health professionals don't feel confident they can meet the needs of both parties.

I recognise that these reactions from health professionals are about their clients and trying to do the best for them; they are not about health professionals trying to look after themselves. Importantly, successful interventions in manual handling can involve taking some kind of risk. Risk is not always bad – yet we have convinced ourselves that it is. We need to connect with the emotions we feel about taking risks with our clients and their carers, and be truthful with ourselves about whether fear is holding us back. We can't escape fear; we can only transform it into something we can live and work with for the positive gain of our clients and their carers.

* * *

I believe manual handling is both a science and an art. In this chapter we have highlighted some of the challenges for health professionals looking at these two broad elements. Now let's look at how these translate to the assessment process itself.

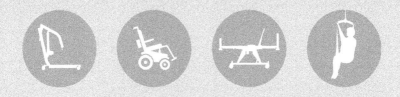

Part II

The challenges with the assessment process

This part first outlines some of the challenges with the assessment in achieving a safe and efficient manual handling routine. I then look at the risk assessment process as the way in which we solve manual handling problems and ask whether focusing on safety is enough. Finally, I explore more of the missed opportunities we could experience by stopping at safety in solving manual handling problems.

Let's stop overplaying the WHS card

I recently assessed a 94-year-old client who was completing slide board transfers from her chair to her bed and back with the assistance of her 91-year-old husband. He was starting to find this transfer really difficult and so her care worker was required to do these transfers. I was called in by the care worker's agency to prescribe a hoist.

This client did not want to use to a hoist. She'd had a bad experience of using a hoist while in hospital, was adamant she wanted to continue to do slide board transfers and felt she was able to do so.

I completed an assessment of her transfer and confirmed that she did not have the skills to do the slide board transfer. This was quite obvious to everyone except for her. This client was exceptionally motivated. She had a standing frame in her house where she would do exercises daily. She had been given a rehabilitation program and she was sticking to it. The lying to sitting transfers were a significant problem also, however, even with a height-adjustable bed, meaning a full lifting hoist was the only option.

Allied health professionals have two options in this kind of situation. We can force clients to comply with a new transfer regime or we can facilitate them coming to the conclusion they need to when they are ready.

For WHS reasons you must …

I realised very quickly in my role as a manual handling advisor that I had a lot of power. The WHS agenda ruled and I could essentially go into a client's home and play the WHS card, demanding that they cease doing a certain transfer they were doing. I didn't really need to explain or justify this demand – if the care worker was unsafe, everything had to change.

By playing this WHS card, we are essentially saying to the client that they need to do something for 'WHS reasons'. The care worker is at risk of being injured and so, if they still want a service, they need to comply with our needs to make the care worker safe or else they lose a service. The 'something' they have to change, in many incidences, is the way they are assisted with the most private aspects of their lives and the way they are moved during these activities.

While we can achieve the outcome of the care worker being safe, let's examine what else happens when we play the WHS card. If we say this, we are going to get our desired outcome. The client is likely to say yes, they will make this change and we will get them to agree to whatever demand we put in place. While this is not meant to be a threatening interaction, it is essentially blackmail, because the client will lose care if they don't do what they are being asked to do.

For the client mentioned at the start of this chapter, part of playing the WHS card would have involved lecturing her about how she needed to use a hoist to keep everyone safe and, in her particular case, highlighting that her husband couldn't continue to lift her like he was. In other words, I could have lectured her in things she probably already knew. I could have made her feel more guilty and selfish than she probably already felt. If I had done this, I would have crushed her dreams and aspirations, and belittled everything she had diligently worked towards over the previous year.

When we use a demand like this, we take control away from the client – and in the place they feel the safest – their home, their castle. Control is a really important human need, and taking it away can lead to resentment and anger. These feelings heighten when this happens under a person's own roof.

Care is a partnership between a client and a care worker, and this partnership can commonly create exceptionally strong bonds and long-lasting friendships. Some care workers have reported to me, however, that their relationship with the client has never fully recovered after a 'WHS card-playing' situation. In this way, and as mentioned earlier in this book, care workers have explained to me that allied health professionals and manual handling advisors can solve a *manual handling* risk but replace it with a *stress* risk.

Situations like this can completely fracture a trusting bond, especially if the care worker was the one who originally submitted a hazard. As clinicians, we make recommendations, write a report and then discharge a client. The care worker has to go into that client's home the next day, and every day after that. Implementing new recommendations can create an exceptionally challenging workplace for the care worker. As I have also mentioned earlier, anxiety and stress is the highest occupational disease in NSW and care workers have the greatest number of stress claims by occupation[1].

---

1   Workcover (2012/13). 'Statistical bulletin 2012/13' NSW workers compensation statistics. Retrieved 8 August 2017 from www.opengov.nsw.gov.au/download/14319.

... Or we can try it a different way

So what can we do differently? If we frame this change in grief, we can start to understand what is going on using a different lens. The stages of grief developed by Elisabeth Kubler-Ross over 30 years ago include denial, anger, bargaining, depression and acceptance[2]. Using a model such as this highlights the number of emotions a person goes through when they are grieving about something.

As clinicians, we are trained in assessing client needs. We see disability all the time and so quickly know when a client might need this item of equipment or need to change what they are doing. In many instances, however, the client doesn't know. While we do this kind of assessment all the time, they are doing this for the first time.

Secondly, while a person may know something cognitively, they might not be ready emotionally to accept it. This is where people can go into emotional denial, because admitting something to themselves means they can't go back. Acceptance is a massive emotional step to make. The reality and acceptance of this outcome is something that can be really hard to come to terms with.

A massive oversight in playing any WHS card and when working through the subsequent stages in that process is to completely ignore the emotions the client might be going through. If we have a framework for addressing these emotions and doing so in a timely fashion, we can achieve care worker safety but also keep the client in control as much as possible. We have the potential to achieve a win–win solution for all parties and avoid ongoing assessment creep – without replacing a manual handling risk with a stress risk.

---

2   Kubler-Ross, E. (2014). On Death and Dying: What the Dying Have to Teach Doctors, Nurses, Clergy and Their Own Families. Scribner: New York.

Re-thinking our use of risk assessment

Risk assessment is the process we use to solve manual handling problems. In my clinical practice and teaching in mental health, I had to both study risk assessment and apply it to practice. Similarly, when my clinical practice and my teaching (through my courses) were more focused on manual handling, I also had to study risk assessment and apply it in practice.

Although risk assessment is performed in exactly the same way, essentially using the same framework, we use it differently in mental health and manual handling. As I will explain in this chapter, in mental health, we get double the use out of it while in manual handling we use it once. I think we can apply a lot from the mental health literature and risk assessment process to manual handling – and we can achieve some great outcomes for our care workers, our clients and for ourselves as allied health professionals if we do.

What is risk management?

Let's start with being really clear on what risk management (and then risk assessment and risk control) is. Risk management is a problem-solving process that involves identifying a problem, assessing it and then putting an action plan in place to solve the problem.

In other words, as the following figure shows, risk management is a three-part process of identifying, assessing and controlling risks.

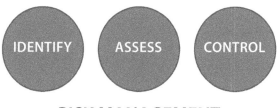

RISK MANAGEMENT

What is risk assessment?

Risk assessment is the second step in the risk management process. Risk assessment is the process of assessing the outcome of risk and how likely this is to occur, and then outlining what action is required based on this. It also tells us how urgently action is required, through coming up with a score based on the severity of what might happen and the chance of it happening. This is usually set out on a risk matrix.

The following figure shows a standard risk assessment matrix for clinical practice.

	VERY LIKELY	LIKELY	UNLIKELY
HIGH *Serious injury*	1	1	2
MEDIUM *Temporary* *incapacity*	1	2	3
LOW *Inconvenience*	2	3	3

SEVERITY

The numbers in the matrix indicate the action required and when, as follows:

1   Serious situation. Cease immediately.

2   Take action in timely manner.

3   Put a plan in place to address the problem.

So risk assessment is essentially a problem-solving tool, and it is widely used and applied to many different decision-making situations.

What about risk control?

Risk control is the process of managing the risks that presented in the assessment stage. Risk control is communicated in terms of a hierarchy (as seen in the following figure). The top option (eliminate) is the most effective method, with the hierarchy of options then working down towards the least effective option (administrative control). Multiple levels on the hierarchy can be used simultaneously to minimise a specific risk.

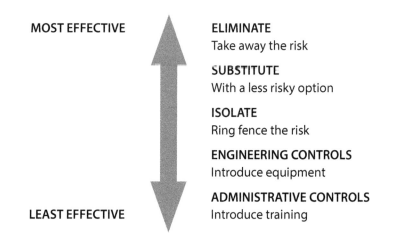

MOST EFFECTIVE

ELIMINATE
Take away the risk

SUBSTITUTE
With a less risky option

ISOLATE
Ring fence the risk

ENGINEERING CONTROLS
Introduce equipment

ADMINISTRATIVE CONTROLS
Introduce training

LEAST EFFECTIVE

But what is risk?

So the essential 'thing' we are trying to manage in this risk assessment process is risk. However, the way risk is defined is where I noticed a fundamental difference across sectors. In the manual handling sector, risk is equated with injury. All our interventions are around preventing back injury. So when you hear the word 'risk' in manual handling, you also hear words such as 'danger', 'injury', 'loss', 'litigation' and 'fear'. Our aim in manual handling is to move from this danger to safety. When we have safety, the risk is gone and we have controlled the risk.

For example, say we have a person who is doing standing transfers but they are not able to weight bear consistently. This means the care worker supporting them is taking a lot of their weight, and that care worker is considered at risk of back injury if things stay the same. We can assume this lift would happen daily, sometimes twice a day. We can also assume that if the care worker did get an injury, it would be serious and likely to cause permanent incapacity. Using the standard risk assessment matrix (introduced earlier in this chapter), we would conclude that because this task is performed twice a day, the likelihood of the risk occurring is 'likely' and, because they are likely to get a serious injury, the severity can be classed as 'high'. This means the risk would be given a measure of 1, with the required action being cease now.

In mental health, risk is defined a bit differently – and in a way that is similar to many other areas of health. We do see the negative words of 'loss', 'injury' and 'danger'. However, we also see other words and phrases sprouting up when we look at mental health, such as 'dignity of risk', 'therapeutic risk-taking', 'gain', 'grow', 'learn' and 'opportunity'.

To give an example, in my work in a crisis mental health team, we would see people in the community who wanted to take their own life. People would usually be brought into the emergency department by ambulance with these thoughts of self-harm. We would have to do a risk assessment in order to preserve their life and determine how likely it was that they were going to go through with that act to take their own life. Essentially, our role was to determine whether this person needed to be admitted to hospital or not in order to preserve their life.

So the severity of the risk here was possible death and the situation would score highly on that side of the risk assessment matrix. The likelihood of this risk occurring was a more complex assessment. We measured this based on a number of key factors (drawn from research), which would indicate how likely the person was to action their thoughts. In this stage, we were looking at moving someone from danger to safety, just as we do in manual handling.

Beyond safety in mental health

Interestingly, in mental health, when we moved the person from danger to safety, we didn't stop there. After someone was determined to be safe, we would take the next step of moving beyond safety to a quality life. This was called 'therapeutic risk-taking' and it involved pushing the boundaries of what people were doing to enhance their quality of life.

When a person's mental health was more stable, we would revisit our risk assessment and use it the opposite way – that is, to test possible activities out. And in this assessment, we would look at the *opportunity* in doing an activity as well as its risks.

We would look at the severity of the risk if something negative happened but also the extent of the opportunity if something good happened. And we would assess the likelihood of something happening to determine whether it was a good idea to assist someone in taking this risk or not. The theory behind this was that these people could stay in hospital for the rest of their lives or we could support them to take some risks and make progress – out of the hospital setting and back into the community. Along the way, we would continue to monitor all risks and opportunities, using risk assessment to keep the negatives in check and enhance the positives. In this way, risk-taking became therapeutic.

This kind of risk-taking is where 'life' is and, as a professional group working with people in these situations, this is where we saw the real magic happening.

Beyond safety in manual handling

Taking this approach of therapeutic risk-taking from mental health, I started to think about whether we could apply a similar approach to manual handling – that is, whether we could consider the opportunity of an activity as well as its risks.

In many of my manual handling assessments, I saw the equipment was in place but the manual handling was still hard for the care worker. I used to try to see if I could be a little creative in the use of the equipment in place to reduce the amount of manual handling a care worker had to do. I started to demand more from the equipment that I was seeing and I started to notice some patterns in the way equipment was used – and when it didn't work as well as it could. I started to notice patterns in the kinds of prescribed equipment that were leading to excessively more manual handling than others.

So, once safe equipment was in place, I started to look at whether we could use risk assessment creatively to investigate the opportunities offered by the equipment, and how much more of the manual handling we could eliminate by making the equipment do the work and not us.

You can use these principles in your educational learning as an allied health professional and when you explore equipment in continuing professional development (CPD) activities. This is not something I advocate using with any client – wait until you are very confident you have completed an exhaustive risk assessment in these learning environments to ensure no dangerous elements prevent you using equipment. This involves engaging with manufacturers in terms of how equipment is being used to do a check on whether contraindications exist to client safety when using equipment in the manner proposed.

Safety is not the end point

Our job as allied health professionals is to advise on safe manual handling routines for our clients and the care workers who support them. However, a safe routine can still be a hard one. The opportunities that exist to go beyond safety and make a manual handling routine safe as well as easy are massive. Our most important role is to aspire to eliminate any possible arduous manual handling routines for our clients and the care workers who support them.

In manual handling, we have assumed that safety is a good outcome – and the end game. We make an assumption that when equipment is in place, a routine is safe and our job is done. With the high-quality equipment we now have available to us, however, we can move beyond safety and risk-reduction to come up with a smooth routine for our clients that increases opportunities and aims for efficiency as well as safety.

Counting all the missed opportunities

As I argue in the previous chapter, risk assessment can be a tool to problem-solve how we can make things happen by both identifying the negative aspects and controlling for them, and enhancing the positive aspects.

Our narrow view of risk assessment (as being all about safety) has many consequences in the work we do in manual handling. This is not only in terms of outcomes for our clients, but also for us as clinicians in loving what we do and achieving some seriously clever problem solving.

Safe with equipment, but what about easy?

Just a couple of months ago, I was asked to assess whether a client needed a two-person service because the care workers were finding this client's care very difficult. She had been prescribed a hoist ten years ago when she became non-weight-bearing, but care workers were now finding positioning the client in the chair really difficult. Upon assessment, I noted a massive pull was needed to position the client back into the wheelchair. When she was lowered into her chair, the hoist fell short of the drop-down point on the chair, which was the back of her chair, by 15 centimetres. This gap meant the care worker had to pull her into the correct position. I prescribed a larger hoist, which meant that the 15 centimetres were eliminated and so the pull into the chair was also eliminated. We were able to prevent this excessive pulling for the next ten years and avoid the unnecessary addition of a second care worker.

A perception exists in manual handling that once you have equipment, everything is solved. Equipment will move a routine from the danger zone to the safety zone. In many incidences, however, equipment will make things safe but still hard. When a care worker and client need to go through routines every day, sometimes twice a day, this hardship builds up to become something that causes exhaustion and a significant reduction in the quality of life. We need to start thinking beyond safety to aim for a quality life possible that is easier, efficient and more tolerable for the client and their care worker. This will, in turn, create a happier client, a more resourceful care worker and a health professional who achieves outcomes that make a real difference.

Sometimes allied health professionals don't see the benefits that the right equipment can make to the manual handling process. In the example I've just given, in the ten years this woman had this equipment, it would have been easy to miss the opportunity to make things easier. Sometimes health professionals neglect many features on the equipment that can enhance care, but they also don't know how to prescribe correctly within a certain range to get the best out of the products.

Driving a Ferrari in third gear?

A massive array of quality equipment is available to us now as allied health professionals to solve manual handling problems. In my teaching and working with health professionals, however, I've noticed a lack of basic knowledge as to how to get the best out of the equipment health professionals are working with, and how to use the full range of the available piece of equipment. Earlier in the book, I equated this to investing in a Ferrari and then driving it in third gear. We have got to start trusting what our equipment can do for us. Allied health professionals need to have the confidence to explore equipment, test it out and see what it can do for them in solving manual handling problems.

Risk assessment to explore

As I outline in chapter 7, we are conditioned in manual handling to do a risk assessment when danger is present. Our aim is to go from danger to safety, and we never really use risk assessment to explore.

Risk assessment is a really clever tool that can ensure that everything we do goes through the safety check. Knowing that this safety check is the grounding of risk assessment, why are we not exploring first and using risk assessment to check? Using a model like this, you can get to know all the attributes your equipment has to offer. You can use the risk assessment to check the safety of using all the available features in particular ways before bringing them into a clinical case. This allows you to start getting to know your equipment intimately and become confident with it.

Let's know when to ditch the rules

Manual handling is full of rules, and rules have a place. They guide care workers into a streamlined routine for their clients without having to make decisions. A care worker's role does not necessarily involve assessment, although I personally think we should be upskilling them in this. Their main role is to 'do' – and to do in the most efficient way possible.

The idea behind using rules in manual handling is that the research would find out the answers as to what way of doing something is the most efficient. Once this most efficient method is found, a rule can be introduced to inform the industry about how to implement this preferred method. This rule is not necessarily something official, but something that filters through the industry via educational seminars and conferences.

From my workshops, I know a significant source of knowledge in these kinds of informal 'rules' is senior colleagues, and I am interested in this source of knowledge. Michael O'Donnell, in *A Sceptic's Medical Dictionary*, suggested that the experience of senior colleagues is not always a great source of knowledge, because 'to many people experience means making the same mistakes with increasing confidence over an impressive number of years'[1].

When I started in the manual handling industry, I was bombarded with all the rules. My problem was I had a shocking memory and I could never remember which rules applied to what. The only way I could remember which rules should be applied was to 'do' and to test. We had an equipment room set up in our office and I used to go in there with my colleagues and explore these rules. I watched seasoned manual handling advisors and saw the way they would test the equipment, and the confidence they had when doing so. Some of the solutions that came out of this were fantastic. I decided I liked this model of experimentation (rather than blind rule-following) and so I took it with me. It was in the 'doing' – and through using the risk assessment process to test out accepted rules

---

1 O'Donnell, M. 1997. *A Sceptic's Medical Dictionary*. BMJ Books.

– that I started to realise what rules made sense and when other rules might be placing limits on us. I am not advocating to ignore rules; I am suggesting you always need to understand why the rule is there.

The most effective way of working out what works best in a particular situation is to feel it. By getting your equipment, outlining your options and using creative risk management as a tool, you can find out the best option for safety and efficiency, and be confident in the decision that you make.

Looking for danger in the wrong place

Safety is non-negotiable in the manual handling space. We are dealing with the movement of people and we need to ensure that the bottom line of safety is always ensured for both the caregiver and the care receiver.

However, I feel rules have a second drawback that can be also quite serious. For example, let's look at the example of brakes on a hoist, and whether they should be on or off when transferring. When I ask this question in my workshops, I see a number of clinicians who feel very anxious about playing around with the hoist's brakes on and off, even in a training scenario. In one recent workshop, one health professional was so anxious about an activity where we experimented with having the hoist's brakes on and off during a transfer that they did not feel comfortable in participating in it. She felt so anxious the hoist would tip in this scenario and did not ever want to take that risk.

Of course, a fall from a hoist is a very serious matter. A fall can result in serious injury or death. From my informal research, falls occur most commonly because the wrong sling has been used or because the sling has not been attached onto the hoist correctly.

When we believe that a hoist can tip through either putting the brakes on or off – a belief perhaps based on the rules that have been handed down to us – we are sourcing our anxiety from the wrong place. We are, therefore, worrying about safety in an area where the risk is low. What is more troubling is that this obsession is deflecting our attention from the place where it matters.

Risk being framed in a negative light in manual handling creates an air of anxiety among allied health professionals. This is paralysing them and stopping them from using the equipment around them to its full potential – that is, this anxiety is stopping them from doing all within their grasp to eliminate manual handling.

Using risk assessment to compare and make decisions

As allied health professionals, we are very good at using risk assessment to confirm something new is wrong, but we are not good at testing the alternative to it to see if it is worse!

All risk assessment results in residual risk – that is, a level of risk that is present no matter how much we try to control it. The Person–Environment–Occupation–Performance model (PEOP) introduced in chapter 1 highlights all the factors that come into play in a manual handling scenario. Our role as advisors is to find and take the lesser of two evils.

Health professionals assume that alternative or new routines are unsafe because they have never tried them. But they don't expose their accepted practices, those they do all the time, to the same level of risk assessment.

In the manual handling sector, when we have a new option to try out, we do a risk assessment on that and we come up with a decision on whether to go with this new option or go with what we 'know'. If the risk of the new option is too high, we go with what we know. We rarely, however, do the risk assessment on the bit we know, so we have no real way of objectively comparing what our old idea looks like in relation to the new idea.

Sometimes you get it in your head that something is unsafe, but then you assess it with an objective eye, perhaps getting colleagues involved, and you realise the risk in this option is actually quite low so why not give it a go. A risk assessment allows you to work that out and justify it.

When I ask allied health professionals how useful they think risk assessments are, I always have a section of the audience who really get it. But another group will argue they are a complete waste of time and really tell me things that are not all that useful. If you're in this second group, you're not using risk assessment correctly. Risk assessment is the cleverest tool when you get to use it right – and it is risk assessment that allows me to feel confident in the recommendations I make.

And remember – sometimes we focus on injury as something that can be controlled, but in doing so we set ourselves up for failure because we can't possibly control it completely. Risk assessment is all about reducing risk while finding opportunity.

In the following part, I draw together all these ideas about using equipment and risk assessment more effectively to outline the ten principles of my manual handling revolution.

Part III

The ten principles

In this part, I outline the ten principles of the manual handling revolution. I think these principles are critical to achieving the outcome of a well-resourced care worker, happy client and confident allied health professional. At the end of each principle, I provide you with some questions to help you start to implement these principles in practice.

The ten principles are:
1. Understand it's a negotiation
2. Address the grief
3. Stop throwing care workers at the problem
4. Manage the manual handling neurosis
5. Use systematic assessment
6. Implement objective guidelines
7. Get creative
8. Use equipment evaluation to separate the gem from the gimmick
9. Consider alternatives to get an outcome
10. Use the assessment guide

Principle 1:
Understand it's
a negotiation

Whatever perspective allied health professionals find themselves representing – that of the person with the disability or the care worker's – the reality is we are dealing with a team. The challenge with working with that team is balancing the needs of the team members when they can seem so much at odds with one another. But when we begin to look more closely at those needs, and at how they can be aligned through negotiation, we start to see some misconceptions.

One of the biggest misconceptions about manual handling is that the care worker and the client want different things. The client wants to be as independent as they can be and the care worker needs to be as safe as they can be. The theory goes that the more independent we push the client to be, the more at risk we place the care worker. The safer we make the care worker, the more restrictions we place on the client. We find when we dive a little deeper into this, however, that the desire for independence and safety aren't actually at odds. Both the client and the care worker often want a lot of the same things. They just may need us to help them see that.

It's a negotiation

I have always been interested in the art of negotiation and how talented people can convince others to come to their way of thinking. Originally published in 1981 (with many subsequent editions), *Getting to Yes: Negotiating Agreement without Giving In* by Roger Fisher and William Ury is a classic guide to negotiation[1]. According to the authors, the aim of any negotiation is to achieve three things:

- a win–win outcome – where both parties feel they have won

- to build a relationship – as opposed to fracture it

- to be efficient – that is, in the way the negotiation achieves this outcome.

However, standard client–care worker conflicts often fail to realise the discussion is a negotiation, and that the preceding three outcomes should be aimed for. A recent case I was involved with highlighted a common type of conflict between a health professional and a care worker. The professional was a therapist offering assistance in a group home for people with complex physical and intellectual disabilities. A client in the group home was being showered on a bath shower trolley when he had the ability to sit up independently and so was a candidate for sitting. The health professional felt it was inappropriate that this client was being washed on this shower trolley, and so suggested to care workers that he should be washed on a shower commode chair instead.

---

1   Fisher, R, Ury, W, & Patton, B. (2011). *Getting to Yes: Negotiating Agreement without Giving In.* Penguin: New York.

The health professional brought the shower commode chair to a meeting so the care workers could get more of a feel for it, and highlighted reasons it was inappropriate for the client to be showered on a bath shower trolley – mainly because it was undignified – and argued that a shower chair should be used. The care workers were very resistant and ended up refusing point-blank to allow this change in procedure. The therapist and the care staff in the group home were then stuck in a massive stand-off, with neither group wanting to back down. In the end, the health professional got a similar outcome as I once did, and she was asked to leave the group home. It was at this stage that I became involved in the case as an independent advisor.

The therapist felt she had genuine concerns for the health and wellbeing of the client, and that they should bring these concerns to a discussion with the care workers. What was missed in this process was the need to address the health and wellbeing concerns of the care workers. If therapists approach an interaction as a negotiation, rather than a situation where they should simply tell the other side what is best for them, they will have a better chance of getting the outcome they seek.

In this situation, through my intervention, I didn't end up recommending the shower commode chair because, through the negotiation, I was able to understand why the care workers were resistant to the chair. These reasons were sufficient to continue with the bath shower trolley. (This will be discussed a little more in chapter 13, which covers systematic assessment.)

Negotiation principles

In *Getting to Yes*, Fisher and Ury outline a negotiation model with four basic principles. When negotiating we need to:

* separate people from the problem

- focus on interests not positions
- insist on using objective criteria
- explore options before deciding what to do.

A model like this can be excellent at bringing up sensitive (but sometimes unacknowledged) topics for the client, family and the care workers, so we get a good outcome for all.

Separating the people from the problem

Fisher and Ury argue we need to be hard on the problem but soft on the people. We need to build a relationship with the various people we are working with. We need to be kind and respectful, and have an appreciation of what they are experiencing. We need to empathise with them. While being kind to the people involved, however, we can be hard on the problem that is before us.

In the example I outlined earlier in this chapter, the therapist did not build a relationship with the care workers. She did not take the time to gain credibility and an understanding that the needs of the staff and the clients are both equally important in processes such as these.

Focus on interests not positions

Fisher and Ury also talk about focusing on interests, not positions in any negotiation. The biggest mistake we make in manual handling is to focus on positions. Positions are what people will say or argue for (or against), and interests are the reasons why they take this position. In the example I outlined, the therapist's position was that shower trolleys should not be used, while the care workers' position was that they should.

Our job as assessors is to understand the 'whys' behind the positions. This can involve asking lots of open questions (what, when, how, tell me). Once we understand the 'whys', we can understand the position taken. Fisher and Ury talk about two things happening when you start to uncover the underlying interests: you will find some interests that are the same and some interests that differ. As an assessor, you can promote the interests that are the same and you can find a way to reframe the interests that are different. Sometimes wanting different things can be seen as a positive.

This is illustrated with the classic example of the two sisters fighting over an orange. The obvious solution would be to divide the orange in two, right? However, when we ask why they want the orange, we might find that one wants the juice and the other the rind. By recognising both of these interests, both can get what they want – a win–win solution.

In the example of the health professional who felt clients should be washed on a shower commode chair, the care workers felt the client should be washed on a bath shower trolley. Instead of getting into loggerheads about positions, we need to fully understand why. We need to spend time on this 'why' to understand the broader context of their interests.

In this example, this involves observing both ways of showering the person using an activity analysis (see chapter 13), and asking the care worker their thoughts. This is an opportunity for the health professional to build a relationship with the care worker and show that the overall wellbeing of the team is paramount. It also allows the health professional to share some tips on how we can make the practice of using the shower commode chair as easy as possible. If the care worker does not find this easier, we need to listen and understand before we ever advise.

In this situation, viewing both transfers allowed me to see why the care workers were adamantly in favour of continuing to use the bath shower trolley. Based on the environment and equipment resources to wash the client, showering on a shower commode chair would have involved two additional transfers. The client was relaxed and happy on the bath shower trolley yet anxious on the shower commode chair. While something looked clear-cut on paper, it was not as clear-cut in practice. Care workers have to do functional tasks for their clients and they need to be able to do this task efficiently.

The argument that ensued over a shower commode chair versus a bath shower trolley meant both the carer and the health professional had entered the 'boxing ring'. Once you go into the boxing ring, it is very hard to get out of it. It can involve both parties becoming even more entrenched in their position because the other side is so opposed to it. It can become a matter of pride and can waste time.

One side may need to back down in this situation, because a decision is going to be made – either for the bath shower trolley or for the shower commode chair. A really important aspect of the process is allowing people to save face.

Options for mutual gain

Fisher and Ury suggest we use a two-stage process for coming up with options and possible solutions. The first stage is freely suggesting options and the second stage is assessing them for viability.

In the situation with the shower trolley versus the shower commode chair we needed to get together as a team and put options on the table. Without judging any of these options in terms of whether they will work or not, we needed to come up with a list of options where everyone felt they had been heard. I could then support the team with assessing these options for viability.

Objective criteria

Next, Fisher and Ury suggest that every decision should be made based on objective criteria. People want an outcome to be fair and reasonable, and an objective measure provides something other than opinion to make this decision. As discussed in chapter 18 (principle 10), all parties need to be aware of this before the assessment begins. An objective measure is some kind of official assessment measure, policy or research finding that guides what is correct practice. The more official that measure can be, the better. With something like this providing a benchmark for all decisions, we are more likely to keep focused on the problem, allowing us to be soft on the people.

Continuing with the example, I was objectively able to conclude that staff wellbeing and client wellbeing were better served by showering on the bath shower trolley. I was also able to use the policy of the organisation to support this decision.

Principle 1 summary

Manual handling is a team-based activity. At times, we need to negotiate to ensure the needs of these team members are met.

The aim of negotiation is to achieve win–win outcomes, build a relationship and be efficient in the way this is done.

Be hard on the manual handling problem, but soft on the people around it.

- Recognise interests lie behind positions. Seek to ask lots of open questions (what, tell me, when, how) to find out these interests.

- Allow all parties to come up with solutions to the problem. Separate the task of coming up with options from the task of assessing the practicality of an option.

- Aspire for decisions to be made based on transparent, objective criteria. Seek to ensure that all parties are aware of these objective criteria before the assessment begins.

Activities

- Think about a case that involved these social and emotional elements of manual handling.

- What were the positions of both parties and what interests lay behind the positions they were taking?

- How could you have implemented Fisher and Ury's four principles of negotiation to efficiently and effectively address the needs of both parties?

10 Principle 2: Address the grief

The introduction of manual handling to a person's life means they are losing something. This loss can be a significant transition for the person as they come to terms with losing their independence.

As assessors or health professionals balancing the needs for independence for the client with the health and safety of the care worker, we can often feel that either the client or care worker is going to get the raw end of the deal. With risk of injury being a more acute matter, the needs of the care worker can sometimes take priority. If we don't implement this change in the right way, we can end up bullying the client. If we get it right, however, we can build a relationship.

In my role as a manual handling advisor, I saw a 13-year-old client with cerebral palsy. She had been seen by our service a number of times in the past, and I recall being told by another therapist that her parent, who was her main caregiver, was really challenging to deal with – in fact, she was described as 'demanding', and she had made a number of complaints in the past after our service was involved. I was asked to assess the manual handling routine because the question was raised again as to whether it was safe for the care worker to assist with standing transfers. The agency felt she needed to use a full lifting hoist.

When I went into the home to do that assessment, the client's parent was exceptionally cold to me and somewhat aggressive. As a health professional, I felt as soon as I saw this client do her first transfer that she needed to use a hoist. She was not able to weight bear and so the care worker was lifting her.

I could see her parent was experiencing an exceptional amount of unresolved grief and this was coming out in anger. Eight years after I did this assessment, I became a parent myself and I now feel I completely underestimated that grief for her. I did not appreciate the relentlessness coupled with immense love that is being a parent – let alone what that is like when your child has a disability. But, even with my lack of this life experience, I was able to recognise and understand some of this parent's grief.

In this situation, I could have used the WHS card and demanded the client use a hoist. I didn't do that. I decided I needed to take another approach and address some of this grief for her parent.

The following sections show how Fisher and Ury's four nego-tiation principles can be applied to a manual handling situation, and I use this example of working with this client and her parent throughout them. While I did involve the client directly during the assessment process and the discussions about options, here I focus on the communications with her parent.

Separating the people from the problem

As outlined in the previous chapter, in *Getting to Yes* Fisher and Ury suggest framing a situation in terms of the problem and not the people in it. In this situation, we could talk about the problem in terms of 'the transfer'. When you separate the problem from the person, you can be as hard as you like on the problem. You then balance that on being soft on the person or people involved.

The skill of being soft on the people is something that has gotten many clever negotiators what they are aiming for. It is a process of building a therapeutic relationship with your client, and fast. We can use these same skills in our work in manual handling, and we need to do so efficiently.

Using people's names

In *How to Make Friends and Influence People* (published in 1935), Dale Carnegie[1] talked about the power of a name. It is the first voice command that, from about 7 months old, we associate with. Someone's name, and the way it is pronounced, is an important part of their identity. Take time to know someone's name, pronounce it correctly and use it. Using someone's name is like fairy dust – it makes people visible, and is a fast way of showing genuine respect and connecting. It changes the landscape for the positive from wherever it otherwise would have been.

In times of conflict, using someone's name can bring the conflict down a notch. In times when a person is going off the point, using names can get them back on track. Even when delivering bad news, using a person's names softens this news.

Many people in my negotiation courses describe feeling sleazy when using peoples' names. Practise this skill in low-stake situations and you will soon get the feel for when you are 'overegging the pudding' and how to get the balance right.

---

1   Carnegie, D. (2010). *How to win friends and influence people*. Ebury Publishing: London.

Asking the magic question

In manual handling, there are times when we have to essentially take control out of someone's hands. Since manual handling now involves two people, we have to take the needs of the two people into consideration, especially when there is a significant risk of injury. In the example previously outlined, the personal care routine involved a lift. Studies have shown that a lift has a high likelihood of causing an injury. I could highlight that risk outright, or I could identify it indirectly. I think in situations like this, you can acknowledge the risk in a way that shows you are clear on the boundaries, but you are being as soft on the person as you possibly can be. You can ask, like I did, the magic question: '[name] tell me one thing I can do for you today that will make this easier on you.'

This question says that you see this person as an individual because you have used their name. It acknowledges this is hard but that you both have to do this. And it creates a pact where the client can take back some control in a situation where they have traditionally had no control.

For the client's parent, this was a pivotal question when asked at the right stage of the assessment process. I asked this when the options that we agreed to explore together did not work out. I knew that was hard for her and I wanted to tell her that I respected how hard that must be.

Establishing the look and connection

Susan Gallagher, in a recent presentation on bariatric care, talked about 'the look' – a connection between two people that acknowledges some kind of understanding[2]. This look can solidify trust,

---

2 Gallagher, S. (2017). 'Taking the first steps in overcoming bias: sensitivity, compassion and the obese patient'. Paper presented at the Bariatric Management Innovation Seminar Series, Concord Hospital, Sydney, Australia, 8 February 2017.

and with the solidification of that trust, we then need to check in with the person that we are honouring this trust. This can be a subtle look at the person's face throughout an assessment process or actually asking them how they are doing.

Focusing on interests not positions

As I outline in the previous chapter, interests are essentially the 'why' behind a stance or position someone takes. Getting back to the earlier example from this chapter, the parent said she didn't want her daughter to use a hoist in her house. This is a position. Positions versus interests can be likened to what you can see of an iceberg versus everything that you can't see beneath the surface. The position is what you can see or what people say. The interests are all the underlying reasons they have for that position. As a negotiator, it is important to know what these interests are. You don't have to agree with them, you just have to hear them.

Finding out interests still requires you to manage the conversation through active listening and having clear time limits.

Active listening is a way of demonstrating that we have heard and have taken on board something a person has to say. You can achieve this through:

- *Paraphrasing:* This is where you repeat back what you hear, changing the words around a little. For example, 'So, it is really important to you for your daughter to be as independent as she can be and reach her goals. Continuing standing transfers is a really important part of that for you.'

- *Reflecting:* This is where you add an emotion onto the paraphrasing. For example, 'So, it is really important to you for your daughter to be as independent as she can be and reach her goals. Continuing standing transfers is a really important part of that for you. It sounds like you would do anything for her.' (You then leave a pause for the other person to respond.)

- *Summarising:* This is where you sum up the main points and then redirect. For example, 'So, it is really important to you for your daughter be as independent as she can be and reach her goals. Continuing standing transfers is a really important part of that for you. It sounds like you would do anything for her. [Name], what manual handling equipment have you guys tried before to reach these goals and what was your experience of that?' *(Redirect.)*

When you put an emotion onto people's experience for them, they can get very emotional. In manual handling, we can sometimes be afraid of emotion and don't know what to do with it. When working in the crisis mental health team, I would see people at the worst time in their lives – when they made the decision they wanted to end their lives. That decision always had a reason behind it, along with immense emotion. In our one-hour assessment, we have to be able to find out the story, hear the emotion, deal with that emotion and come up with a plan. I became very skilled at listening, processing with the person and moving onto a plan.

Aggression is a common emotion and the tendency can be to discipline someone for being verbally aggressive (involving shouting abuse). Often when someone shouts at us, it can feel right to retaliate by raising your voice back at the person. With an intervention like this, you again enter a boxing ring. Once in the ring, you are very unlikely to be able to get out of it and you lose sight of your goal in the intervention. A former colleague of mine described to me how anger could be depression expressed a different way. If we label anger as an emotion, we can follow the active listening guidelines while naming it – for example, '[Name], you sound really angry and frustrated right now'. This way we are more likely to open the streams of communication and start to understand the interests behind the position being verbalised.

Summarising (and redirecting) allows you to keep control of the conversation – because when you open Pandora's box, you need to be able to control it. I published a study recently with occupational therapists in a primary care setting, looking at the barriers to addressing mental health concerns in this setting[3]. The occupational therapist participants in the study stated that they didn't have the time to be able to address mental health concerns along with everything else they had to deal with because it took so much longer to try to solve the client's problem. The key when hearing concerns such as these is that you don't have to solve the problem, you just need to hear it. Solving it might be another service in terms of processing what is happening for the person, but the person providing that service may not be you.

Using these skills, I was able to open the streams of communication between the client's parent and myself. She described the heartache of her journey up to that point and the constant fight she had to advocate for her daughter. She described feeling bullied by services where no-one listened to her or her daughter and what they needed. I was able to use my active listening skills to show her I heard and I understood her position.

Looking at options for mutual gain before deciding what to do

Once we determined that the transfer was unsafe in the manner in which it was being done, the next step was coming up with alternatives, or options for mutual gain. This step involves giving control to the client, family and care worker by asking them what they would like to try. While you may have a clinical hunch that

3   Gallagher, A, Lyons, B, Houston, C, & Cummins, M. (2016). 'Exploring the current and potential role for occupational therapists in managing depression in primary care settings: Perspectives on occupational therapists in Ireland'. *Irish Journal of Occupational Therapy*, 44(2), p 10–18.

something will or will not work, in my 15 years of practice I have been proven wrong many times. The client is an expert in their own situation, so it is important for the client to lead this. I do give my honest opinion but still facilitate the client to have input by saying something like, 'I don't think this will work, but I would love to be proven wrong, so let's try it and see'. As outlined in chapter 9, it is important to keep the process of coming up with solutions separate from the process of assessing them. Giving this control is another aspect of building a relationship based on trust, because you are showing you respect the views of the client.

In this situation, the client's parent and I agreed to trial various standing transfer aids to see if they could reduce the strain on the care worker. At best we may have come up with a solution that could work beautifully; at worst, it could help the client and her parent to process the conclusion themselves.

Using objective criteria

As discussed in chapter 9, Fisher and Ury talk about using objective criteria and I think this is a key aspect of manual handling interventions. You need to have some way of showing your clients that the decisions you make, which may not be popular, are based on some objective measure. Remember – we are often in the business of giving bad news in our role as health professionals in manual handling, and we need to be able to outline why this bad news is objectively required.

Objective measure for assessment

For this client, I was able to show the client's parent the policy under which I was working as a manual handling advisor (see chapter 14 for more on this). This provided a standard by which to assess options we were trialling as alternatives to a full lifting hoist. This also allowed me to provide something external to me that explained the reasons and allowed me to safely get the client's parent involved in evaluating options for the decisions I needed to make.

In this initial part of the assessment, the objective measure showed what the agency deemed unsafe with manual handling transfers and what we all needed to do to work together to remove risk from the service. The second part of the assessment allowed me to have a measure by which options were assessed so we could decide – together and objectively – whether they passed the criteria for a safe transfer.

Objective measure for time

We can be objective in the way we use time also. By putting a time limit on conversations before we start a discussion, the client is aware of how much depth they are going to go into in this conversation. This gives them a marker of the level of detail we want them to convey, and allows them to start gearing their story to fit into that time frame.

For example, you can start the conversation by saying something like, 'I wanted to talk to you for about five minutes about your experience up to now with transfers and how the assessment process has been for you so far.'

The client knows it is a brief conversation, not an hour-long counselling session. It gives them the marker that they need to tell you as much as they can in that five minutes so they give you the key points. The five minutes allows you to summarise with confidence and respect to ensure you get all relevant information in the five minutes. You can always give more than five minutes but you can rarely give less. Without this five-minute marker before you start, however, it can turn into a 20-minute ramble. So, whatever time you have, always set it. Then you can confidently and respectfully change the conversation where you need to.

Again, in manual handling, your role is to assess manual handling tasks and come up with a solution. That has many emotional elements. Your role is to know them and acknowledge them. You can redirect people on where they can get extra help if they need to deal with any distress.

When you use objective measures for assessment and your time, you can be as hard as you want about the problem while remaining soft on the people.

Using these principles in the scenario explained through this chapter, I was able to develop a strong therapeutic relationship with the client's parent as well as with the client. Using the trust established with them in a short time, I was able to guide them through the assessment process. We tried a number of standing transfer aids, identified by both the client and the client's parent. Although they didn't work, being open to trying something on their terms was very important to them.

You may question if it is an efficient use of time to try options that you have a strong clinical justification for believing will not work. Giving clear guides in terms of time allocations outlined in chapter 18 (principle 10), you can manage expectations to result in an efficient and effective process. Our aim is to complete a comprehensive assessment to avoid assessment creep – that is, a situation where the assessment goes on long after the face-to-face part has taken place.

In the example I have given, we ended up collaboratively concluding that a hoist was needed, and so a hoist was put in place in the family home. While this was still a challenging process for the client and her parent, I was able to be with them through that journey (which had to happen) and identify the supports available to them. I was confident that by just attempting to walk a mile in the shoes of the parent and her daughter during the assessment process, I was able to empathise with the both of them and, therefore, provide a positive outcome to what could have been considered a negative intervention.

Principle 2 summary

Grief can be a significant factor in manual handling. It can display itself along a spectrum of emotions from anger to apathy.

You will never win an argument. When someone wants to go into the boxing ring with you, you have two ways to respond. Stay out of it and your outcome for the wellbeing of that client and their care worker always stays in sight. Go in and you completely lose sight of the goal.

Being soft on the person can involve using their name regularly in conversations, asking the 'magic question' and connecting via a look.

Finding out what someone's interests are involves asking open questions, but also being ready with high-level skills in active listening (paraphrasing, reflecting, summarising) to know what to do with what you have heard.

Look for options for mutual gain. How are interests the same? How are they different?

Objective criteria can be a powerful way to take the personal out of decisions, as you objectively outline decision-making criteria.

Activities

- Rate how good your skills are in the following areas (using 1 for Terrible and 10 for Remarkable):
  - Remembering peoples' names
  - Using peoples' names
  - Asking clear, open questions (where, what, tell me, how, when)
  - Using paraphrasing to communicate you are listening and understanding
  - Using reflecting to place an emotion on what you are hearing
  - Using paraphrasing to keep control of the conversation
  - Asking people what they need
  - Using time to set expectations on conversations
  - Using objective measures to set expectations on what is and is not possible

- Pick your three lowest performing items.

- How could you increase your skill level by 10 per cent in each of these three this week?

Principle 3: Stop throwing care workers at the problem

We live in the age of innovation. Advances are being made all the time in terms of assistance technology in addressing manual handling problems. Despite these equipment advances, however, we still have the mentality in the manual handling sector of thinking about more care workers before we look at equipment. I think we have had such low expectations of equipment in the past, we just accept that equipment can be inadequate, when this is not the case. The question about whether a manual handling service should be a one- or two-person service is a question I am asked all the time at the conferences and workshops I present at.

What do we think we are gaining with the second care worker? I have had the opportunity to observe hundreds of personal care routines and I am regularly intrigued about what the second care worker does. I find that sometimes the second care worker is required because of the underutilisation of equipment or the incorrect prescription of equipment.

We are conditioned in manual handling to think that two care workers are 'safer' than one. Purely in terms of workers, we assume that all is better with two. A review by the University of New South Wales in 2013[1] discusses how the research is mixed. While a number of studies show that two care workers have a positive impact on safety, others found that they don't, and the guidelines for avoiding MSI among care workers do not indicate that injuries occur when staff work alone.

Recognising the conflicting evidence, we need to be able to compare the additional challenges introduced to a manual handling routine through an additional person. While we do create an expanded workforce, this also results in a number of consequences that may diminish the labour created. When we are making a decision on whether a second care worker is of merit, we need to be able to objectively compare two care workers with one care worker. As discussed in chapter 7 when outlining the risk assessment process, we need to compare the proposed innovation with the next best alternative.

Sometimes a second care worker is put in place without a full understanding of why the routine is a problem. Without this understanding, we can be exposing two care workers to the same risk faced by one.

Messing up the dance

Observing highly skilled care workers assist a person with a disability is like watching a highly skilled dance, such as a tango. This was the first thing that struck me when I was beamed into my first

---

1 Kayess, R, Valentine, K, Thompson, D, Meltzer, A, & Fisher, KR. (2013), 'Research on the need for two care workers in a community setting: Final report', UNSW Social Policy Research Centre, for Ageing, Disability and Home Care, Department of Family and Community Services NSW. Retrieved 8 August 2017 from www.sprc.unsw.edu.au/media/SPRCFile/Report5_13_TwoCareWorkers_Final_for_web_June_2013.pdf.

manual handling advisor role, knowing nothing about the industry. The speed, care and precision of a partnership at work were incredible. The freedom created was inspiring, even though there was significant disability involved. It was like the energy channels were open. The client worked with the care worker in whatever way they could and the care worker read the cues of the client. I realised this was a very intimate process that can take some time to create. On many occasions, it is never really reached, but even a glimpse of this is of value.

When you introduce another care worker into the mix, the whole dynamic changes. The care workers and client now have to decide on a new dance. They need to learn this new dance in terms of speed, tempo, moves, flow and energy efficiency. They need to be able to apply it to their practice every day and be able to change partners regularly. This is by no means impossible, but it is a more complex process to create and to get right than with just having one care worker with their client. It involves coaching and training. Every element in this is moving and flowing, and if it is missing or out of rhythm, the flow of the dance is interrupted. And every element that is out diminishes the value of that second care worker.

The communication

One key element of this dance is communication, where care workers give and receive cues on when to move, how to move and at what velocity to move. When one care worker is involved, this communication happens between the client and the care worker, usually in the process of making eye contact, using a certain touch or issuing a clear directive.

When there are two care workers involved, the leader needs to communicate with two people. As Kayess and colleagues[2] suggest,

2   *ibid.*

communication gets a little more complicated. The leader needs to manage the eye contact, the touch and the direction. As you can see from the following figure, purely by the physical setting and positioning of everyone involved, the care workers are likely to communicate together because they have closer eye contact. Having to look downwards to meet the client's eye means, more often than not, the client is likely to be left out. With the client unable to participate as much as before, the care workers are likely to need to do more.

Care worker 1   **Care worker 2**

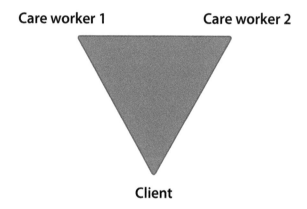

Client

Height of the care worker

In achieving this dance, anthropometrics play a part in certain activities. A key reason a second care worker is usually needed is for rolling on the bed. Rolling on the bed requires the bed at a certain height for the roll to be completed comfortably by the care worker. If the care workers are of two different heights, this can mean one care worker is required to squat significantly to match the height of the second care worker. This can lead to challenges of fatigue for the taller person.

Organisational issues and costs

Providing care in the community is a whole different beast from providing care in the hospital setting. Basically, it is an administration nightmare. An administrator has to schedule two care workers to be in the same place at various specific times throughout the day, balancing the needs of a number of different clients. In terms of geography alone, the challenges quickly become apparent. The biggest challenge in the community is that each client lives in a separate home and the care worker has to go to that home. This means they have to tackle many unknowns in terms of traffic, parking and keeping to a tight schedule.

If a care worker is delayed on any one job during the day, the schedule for the day is adjusted slightly. If the care worker is dealing with a list of clients by themselves, they communicate with the client about the delay and the client has to wait. While this is not a great outcome, only one stream of clients is affected.

Applying this scenario to a situation with two care workers assisting a client, the implications are quite different. If a care worker is late, they don't just have to let their clients know of the delay but also another member of staff. This second member of staff, who was on time for their daily schedule, is now delayed. This means that the stream of clients they are working with throughout the day is now delayed. If one of these clients is a two-person service as well, another care worker's schedule is brought into the mix. The impact of a delay from one stream of care expands exponentially to place the whole system into disarray.

While this has administration costs, it also has end user costs. A two-person service requires two people to be present, so the service cannot start until the two members of staff are present. If a care worker is late by 10 minutes three times per week that equates to $30 per week, because this involves 10 minutes at the start of each service and 10 minutes at the end because they would have to stay to make up for the time. We are now paying for two care workers, so that doubles to $60. Over a year that is more than $1,500 per client per care worker, so if they have two care workers, they're now paying $3,000 extra per year for the highly likely event where a care worker might be a little late. This is just 10 minutes three times per week.

The elephant in the room – the family

Behind many episodes of care in the community is a family who need assistance from a care agency to be able to cope with the role of caring. These people do the caring when the professional care workers are not there. While the agency may provide two care workers, rarely does the family have two members to assist with caring. I find it really frustrating that this is rarely part of the thinking when assessments are completed in terms of care.

While the family may get four hours of care every day, the day has another 20 hours of care when the family are required to support this person. Of course, some services require two people no matter how fantastic an equipment solution you put in place. I see all too often, however, that two people are put in place unnecessarily to make up for ineffective or underutilised equipment. In these cases, the allied health professional has been unable to recognise when an item of equipment is ineffective because they lack the key skills to do so.

I find it heart-wrenching that family members are subjected to performing a significant amount of manual handling per day that could have been avoided if the right equipment was put in place. On many occasions, the family member is the second caregiver and therefore is required to do the care independently when the care worker is not there. Much of this equipment that could cut down on their manual handling is not revolutionary but simple items of equipment that people with disabilities use daily. Not only are the family losing out in terms of excessive manual handling but, with the addition of a second carer, their fee also doubles overnight or the care reduces. This results in the burden of care being placed right back on the family, leading to burnout and stress.

Masking the real problem – equipment fit

In my clinical work, I get referrals for clients where all the equipment is in place but the service is still hard. The request is normally to assess for a second care worker. I recall doing an assessment for a client in her fifties with multiple sclerosis who was fully dependent. She had been prescribed a full lifting hoist ten years previous. The presenting problem was positioning in the shower commode chair and wheelchair.

Through my assessment, I saw the care worker was completing an excessive amount of pulling to position the client into their wheelchair. The service was safe on paper but it was hard. The reason for this pull was simply that the hoist was too small. I prescribed a larger hoist, which allowed the client to reach the correct drop-down point in the chair. This allowed the hoist to do the work of positioning the client in the chair with the care worker only needing to work the controls and do a slight adjustment at the end of the transfer. What was troubling to me was that two manual handling assessments had taken place in that ten-year period. Neither of the assessors had picked up this opportunity, as it can easily be missed if we don't know what we are looking for. Through prescribing the larger hoist now, we were able to delay the need for a second care worker.

This client received four services a day from a private agency equating to 4 hours per day, or 28 hours a week. If each hour is costed at $30, that equates to $840 per week and $43,680 per annum, not taking into consideration penalty rates for work on a weekend and public holiday. If a second care worker went in because of that positioning problem in the chair, which was eliminated by the right hoist, we would have ended up spending $43,680 per annum more on this client. Assuming she lives for another 20 years, which is likely, we saved $873,600 through one simple intervention.

What was also interesting in this case is that the family had to assist the client around this. This meant that if we had introduced two care workers, the family would not only have to pay $873,600 more but would also have had to continue to take the load of the person themselves outside this time, where a simple risk could have been avoided.

The equipment we now have available is in most cases adequate (or more than adequate). Only when equipment is matched and prescribed correctly should we then look at a second care worker. There is no room in 2017 for ineffective equipment in manual handling. Too much excellent equipment is out there to tolerate this. We need to know what correct prescription looks like.

If we are going to conclude that a second care worker is needed, we need to be sure the drawbacks in terms of messing with the dance, anthropometrics and organisational issues are merited by the benefits a second care worker might bring to the situation. The best method of doing this is by completing a risk assessment and comparing your solution to the next best alternative.

The lack of this comparison can leave us recommending interventions that are actually more hazardous than the risk we first sought to solve.

Here are some tips and tricks to avoiding having to prescribe a second care worker:

- Make sure you are getting the best out of the equipment first.

- Check to see if other equipment options could fill the gap. Do a cost benefit analysis of the cost of the equipment and the possible cost involved of a second carer.

- Think about the broader tasks the client needs help with. Do these also merit another person?

- Do the two-person test – are the drawbacks of introducing the second care worker merited for the risk they are solving? Consider the alternatives that might be available (see chapter 17 (principle 9) for more on this).

Checklist before introducing a second care worker

Run through the following before recommending a second care worker:

- Does all your lifting equipment meet pick-up and drop-down points during the transfer routine of your client, without care worker intervention?

- Are you (and the care workers) getting the best use out of all the resources on the equipment?

- Is the care worker correctly using the equipment in place?

- Have you explored equipment options to determine how they might reduce exposure to manual handling?

You might need a second care worker in the following circumstances:

- rolling on the bed if rolling devices are not effective

- positioning in the chair even though drop-down and pick-up points are achieved with lifting equipment

- moving hoist on the floor surface if pivoting the hoist is not appropriate

- uncontrolled movement and extensor spasms where specialist slings that support uncontrolled movements are not effective

- behavioural difficulties that mean you cannot predict a client's behaviour in positioning

- client anxiety in hoisting

- overall number of tasks in the routine is more efficiently completed with two people.

Principle 3 summary

Manual handling is a dance with a communication and energy flow between the care worker and the client.

As a result of reducing resources and increased costs, we should be aspiring for caregiving with one staff member where possible.

When a second care worker is needed, we have to ensure they can tap into that communication and energy flow.

Second care workers are sometimes prescribed because of ineffective equipment or lack of knowledge of equipment options available.

We need to ensure the needs of the family outside of formal care are catered for in manual handling solutions.

Activities

Think about clients you have assessed where two people were assigned. Why do you think this second care worker was needed? Were there potential equipment solutions that could have reduced the need for the second care worker?

Think of three items of equipment that could reduce the number of care workers required for your client

What are your policies and procedures saying about the use of two care workers? Are these merited and why?

Principle 4: Manage the manual handling neurosis

I have been running workshops in manual handling and systematic hoist prescription since 2007. I am always very conscious of the air of anxiety many allied health professionals bring to these events in terms of manual handling. Some health professionals describe living with an almost constant anxiety that someone might get hurt from an intervention they have recommended.

Some health professionals describe hating manual handling and dreading any case that lands on their desk that involves a major manual handling component. One therapist in a negotiation skills workshop I was running described a dreadful situation where therapists became suddenly busy whenever a complex manual handling case came to their desk because they didn't want to take it on.

This anxiety has two main components. The first component comes from assuming they can control much more than they can. The second component comes for the lack of systems to help them justify decisions they have made with the kinds of objective measures that come through comparing it to the next best option they already had.

Let's be clear about what is in our control

When I had my first child, I thought I was an amazing parent. My son slept, he ate and he did what we asked of him (most of the time). *What more would you want?* I thought. This parenting stuff is easy. Then my second son came along, and he did everything but sleep and seemed to mostly throw up instead of eating. He would listen to everything we asked him to do, appear to hear what was being asked, and then do the complete opposite. By the time he was the ripe old age of two, I was clearly getting a lot of grey hairs.

When you are trying to get clients to take on a positive health behaviour, you will get some clients like my first son and some more like my second son. The change you're suggesting makes perfect sense to you – it just may not make sense to them, and they could indeed have a point. After you give advice, they make a decision. This decision can involve changing that behaviour in the way you recommend for positive health gain or doing something other than that. The extent to which you can control that decision is minimal.

A therapist in one of my workshops described an exceptional amount of anxiety after completing a training session in a certain technique with a client's family and care worker. When the therapist went back a couple of weeks later, they found out that the client, the family or care worker were not doing any of the intervention techniques that the therapist had recommended to them. The therapist was experiencing significant anxiety because they felt they would be blamed for not ensuring the client and family undertook the safe intervention recommended.

When I was lecturing, I was advised by my wise mentor that the only thing you can control in lecturing is how you lecture. Teaching is like delivering the post: you don't know what letters are read or even opened. When we teach someone a skill, we have no way of really knowing how much is acquired and retained unless we assess. Equally, after that, we don't know how much they will put into action beyond the assessment process and in the environment where it really matters. We are trying to control the uncontrollable.

A massive amount of manual handling is recognising what is in our control. The level of advice we give is in our control, as is how we give this advice and how we create the best environment we possibly can, so the 'likelihood' of the person taking up the intervention is created. Our aim in manual handling is firstly to identify what is in our control and then to do the best we can at influencing within this space.

Risk assessment is for assessment, not prediction

Risk management language creates a false promise in many ways. The language of 'likelihood' assumes a prediction element and, therefore, seems to indicate our ability to predict behaviour. We have this assumption that just because someone has come into the health service, we should be able to predict their behaviour. This is not always the case; in fact, it is hardly ever the case.

Risk assessment is an exceptional tool in manual handling. It allows us to really nut out what the problem is and how we could come to a solution. Risk assessment is not a prediction tool; it is an assessment tool. We assess with it, rather than predict.

Risk assessment is dynamic

As introduced in chapter 1, the Person–Environment–Occupation–Performance model (PEOP) illustrates all that is at play in any manual handling routine. As allied health professionals, we do a risk assessment to make the best manual handling conclusion possible with the information we have on the risks and opportunities that present themselves.

In my crisis role in mental health, I was working one Saturday with a person who was very unwell. He had a psychotic episode and was living in the community. He was deemed a risk to himself, and the role of our team was to get him to the safety of the hospital so he could get the treatment he needed. When we were assessing him for admission to hospital, he absconded. We worked closely with police, ambulance and his family to determine his whereabouts so we could coordinate admitting him to hospital in the most dignified and respectful way possible.

In my role as a health professional on the crisis team that day, I had to do a risk assessment of the situation to balance the risk he posed to himself against the dignity we needed to show him in bringing him to a safe place. The tricky part was that the details I was basing my risk assessment on kept changing. At 10 am I did a risk assessment and then found, five minutes later, that something had changed – for example, his location – and I would have to revise my risk assessment. Five minutes later again, something else would had changed, such as his erratic behaviour, and I would have to do a risk assessment again to account for that. I learned that day that a risk assessment is out of date the moment you finish it. If one aspect of the situation changes after that risk assessment is completed, the whole situation changes.

We can only do the best we can with the information we have in front of us to make that decision. As clinicians, we have the make a decision and use the best available evidence to do that. Tools like the PEOP model can act as a checklist to help us identify the things that we need to consider in any manual handling routine.

Anxiety in relation to taking risks

In researching for a keynote presentation a number of years ago, I came across Warren Macdonald – an Australian who lost his legs above the knee, after a mountain accident. Following this incident, he continued to mountain climb, and in 2003 he was the first double above-knee amputee to reach the summit of Mount Kilimanjaro. Warren now speaks across the world about resilience and positive risk taking, and a picture of him standing on the top of a mountain in his prosthetics probably perfectly sums up the very reason we became the allied health professionals we did – to allow people to achieve these goals.

I was interested in Warren because he had achieved great things, and I was intrigued by his experience when he told his health professionals in rehabilitation, after losing his two legs, that he wanted to go back to rock climbing. I contacted him and he told me,

> I had a classic situation where I was supposed to learn how to fall in my prosthetics, because it's going to happen, right? And while we have a mat set up in front of me and everything, next thing I've got two health professionals having this conversation, one each side of me, discussing whether we should do this or not. I'm watching this conversation go back and forth, and decided: we're doing it. And I just fell forward. They were kind of freaked, but my thing was, 'What? Are we going to wait and let me fall outside while I'm on my own?'

A massive amount of anxiety can exist among allied health professionals in terms of risk and harm. We can find it difficult to differentiate between good risk and bad risk. We also sometimes find it difficult to justify how doing something like what Warren describes, in terms of letting him fall, is the best thing for him. We then go into conservative risk management where we bury any opportunity to come up with innovative solutions to problems. This scenario explains how we as therapists use risk assessment and the barriers we place on ourselves. If we don't do it, we think, we will be safe. But if we do it, look at how much we could achieve.

Susan Jeffers, author of *Feel the Fear and Do It Anyway*, suggests that the challenges we feel when dealing with fear are based on experience and education – that is, facing anxiety and fear is not primarily a psychological problem, but an educational one.

Making decisions we can feel confident about

An experienced therapist came up to me in the break in one of my workshops, feeling quite anxious after the discussion about standing hoists. She had recommended a standing hoist to a client she just knew in her heart was able for it. Everyone else on the team had opposed the recommendation, so she was on her own in speaking out about it and standing firm on her conclusion. The outcome was that this person was prescribed a standing hoist and was making significant gains with it. The therapist, however, spent the next six months having nightmares about all the things that could happen to that client when using the standing hoist. What if he fell and she was to blame? Everyone else on the team would say, 'You see, we told you' and then she would feel awful about the outcome for this client and his life from then on.

Upon quizzing her on the recommendation she made, she was able to list off a strong argument for the standing hoist. She was able to explain the skills he had that made him a strong candidate for this equipment. She also had a strong justification for not going with a full lifting hoist, explaining many of the impacts on the client and family by going down this route. She explained how she wrote pages in her notes to justify this to herself, and felt she was getting lost in her justification. She was anxious that her notes would not be enough to support her clinical decision and this was what was keeping her up at night.

While this health professional had a strong rationale for making this decision, she didn't have a way in which she could easily prove that to herself and her team around her if anyone was to review her notes. While the argument was there, it was buried in a thesis. Anyone reading this justification would have to decode information to get the key points. In an age where we often have information overload, we need to be able to give a clear justification for decisions such as this – we need to be able to say it in one page. This skill of lean writing is invaluable.

I am really interested in the psychology of decision-making and how you can confirm you have made the best decision you can make. We need a way of controlling our anxiety. People make decisions all the time and the best way of making a decision is to compare our decisions. Fisher and Ury (whose theories on negotiation I introduced in chapter 9 (principle 1)) suggest comparing your answer to the next best alternative, and this can be applied in clinical practice. Using the risk assessment framework I outline in chapter 15, we can do this in manual handling to help us justify clinical decisions to ourselves and all the other stakeholders around us. A key problem is that some of the risk assessment templates we are given to use in our clinical work are of a 'tick the box' nature, and are so disconnected from our everyday decisions that people don't connect the dots.

Residual risk – the lesser of two evils

Residual risk is the 'leftover risk' that remains once we have controlled the risk as far as reasonably practicable. All tasks have residual risk. This is the risk you can't control no matter how much you try. A key thing to remember is that a risk assessment is static and is essentially an attempt at determining what may be advised into the future. By virtue of the fact that we cannot really predict the future with complete assurance, risk assessment in itself is a flawed science. We, therefore, use it to make the best decision we can with the information available to us at that point in time. Sometimes we can feel quite anxious about this level of residual risk, which makes us feel like we should go back into our shell and go with what we have always done.

A really important aspect of risk assessment is the process of comparing. Recognising this residual risk is something we have to work with, we need to determine if this residual risk is acceptable. If not, we need to determine what the next best alternative option is. Essentially, it is a way to check if the option we are assessing is 'the lesser of two evils'.

Application of the next best alternative

I did an assessment for a client in his 50s who had moderate intellectual disability, cerebral palsy and epilepsy. The client had many uncontrolled movements, which increased when he became stressed. The aim in any manual handling procedure is to reduce stress as much as possible. I was asked to assess him because as part of his care he was being bathed, whereas the procedures of the department governing his care said people were not to be bathed due to the risk involved.

While the needs of his ageing parents were important and valid, as an assessor, I needed to know what the bottom line was in terms of care worker safety. If I needed to give the parents bad news, I needed to be able to do that in a way they would understand.

On the outside, this seemed a very straightforward assessment, because bathing involves a lot of bending at a low height and bending was a risk for manual handling injury. In doing this assessment, however, I did two things. Firstly, I observed what he was doing when being bathed and, secondly, I assessed what the alternative would look like. The alternative involved placing him in a shower commode chair over a small level-entry shower in the bathroom.

In bathing, he had a ceiling track hoist to transfer him into the bath. Once in the bath, he sat passively. Washing the side next to where the care worker positioned themselves was easy but washing the opposite side involved a lot of over reaching. How could we reduce the risk from over reaching while washing the opposite side?

The alternative would have involved hoisting the client from bed to the shower commode chair where he would have to sit as opposed to lie. This transfer in itself would not be a problem but the showering would have been. The client had a tendency to grab and, being quite strong, he would pull the care workers. His uncontrolled movements would increase when he was excited or stressed. These uncontrolled movements, although not intentional, were akin to being assaulted and could land a powerful punch.

The client being in the bath created a different scenario. The client really loved the bath and, because of this, he was calmer. Using the shower commode chair, the client would not have the after-effects of calmness for the rest of the day. It was this calmness that helped his ageing parents manage his behaviour.

We came up with the procedure of positioning the client over the bath in the overhead hoist. He would be rotated first so the furthest side was closest to the care worker. They would soap that side when he was at waist height in the overhead hoist. He was then rotated around and placed in the bath like normal. We were able to isolate the risky elements and substitute it with a less risky way of doing it.

What used to really frustrate me about WHS when an action plan was put in place was that no-one assessed this new plan in parallel with the option they were giving up. Sometimes this comparison is really important in helping you as an assessor manage the risks that you just can't and never will be able to control.

Other larger things need to be managed here than just the manual handling risk, yet all these other factors impact the manual handling risk.

We don't always get it right

How we deal with failure is really interesting. Humans overall still have not developed maturity in this space. We treat people terribly who make a mistake and this treatment can potentially ruin their career. In 2007 I had a serious car accident and managed to get out without a scratch. You could do two things with me after such a situation. First, you could never let me drive again because I had crashed a car. Or you could let me drive, knowing I would be a better driver because of the crash – as I know exactly how simply car crashes can happen. I know the feel of them and I know the factors in my behaviour that can cause an accident. With this philosophy, if you let me drive the car again, I am less likely to have a crash because of this heightened awareness.

We have a view that making a mistake is wrong and not making a mistake is right. This philosophy has sent us down a path of conservative risk management and, unless we can free ourselves from this, we are going to stay within the safety zone but eliminate every opportunity to find innovative and creative solutions to problems.

Principle 4 summary

We need to recognise what is in our control in the interventions with our clients. Our role is to advise and help people make the best decisions possible for their health and wellbeing.

Risk assessment is a tool to help users assess manual handling risk. It is not a prediction tool.

We need to be able to divide risk into helpful risk and harmful risk. Our role is to enhance the helpful and minimise the harmful.

Risk will always involve residual risk that remains after a solution is put in place.

A way we can determine which is the best solution going forward is to compare an option to the next best alternative.

Activities

Think about assessments you have been anxious about. Where do you think your anxiety is coming from?

Think about the situation – what is in your control and what is not in your control?

Think about what the next best options were in this intervention. How did they compare to what you recommended?

Principle 5: Use systematic assessment

In my practice as a manual handling advisor, I have assessed many manual handling routines where other professionals were involved before me. Many have achieved exceptional outcomes for their clients while others have not been so successful. On many occasions, a routine may be safe because of the intervention, but I have seen an abundance of cases where opportunities to set up routines efficiently, use equipment to its maximum and eliminate manual handling were missed. A reason for allied health professionals missing these opportunities is the lack of a systematic way of addressing a manual-handling problem. Undertaking any assessment of manual handling involves a system for completing the assessment.

The Person–Environment–Occupation–Performance (PEOP) model (shown again in the following figure) has been used to explain manual handling throughout this book. When we look at this model, it helps us outline the steps to undertaking a manual handling risk assessment to assess for risk that would compromise safety as well as opportunities for efficiencies.

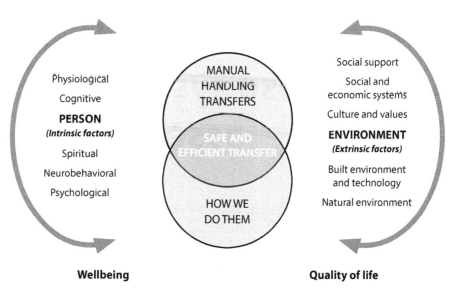

The model has four main components that influence and lead to the outcome of the safe and efficient manual handling routine (or lack thereof). These are:

1   the manual handling transfers – assessed by an activity analysis

2   how we do them – based on objective assessment

3   the impact of the personal factors in how well processes are taking place

4   the impact of the environmental factors in how well processes are taking place.

I outline how these four components come together in the following sections. (Note that my focus here is the activity analysis. More detail on objective assessment is provided in the following principle and chapter.)

Manual handling transfers: Activity analysis

Completing an activity analysis is the backbone of assessing any manual-handling routine; however, it is all too often overlooked. We need to know the steps from start to finish before we are able to comment on it. Each individual step needs to be accounted for. This can mean really breaking the routine down and walking through, step by step, each part with the client and their care worker. The only way of doing this is to observe the real process from start to finish, at the time when it's regularly completed as part of the person's day, in the exact environment in which it takes place. While 'dry runs' are sometimes the only option for doing an assessment, they can fail to fully identify the manual handling issues that might be at play for the client and the care worker supporting them.

Having an activity analysis of what is happening allows us to examine it for opportunities for efficiencies. It also allows us to clearly and objectively assess one routine against another, to make decisions on which routine is safer and more efficient. This, in turn, allows us to clearly and objectively explain our decision-making when advising clients and care workers on the best way of moving forward.

For example, the following activity analysis breaks down all the steps and transfers in a typical morning routine involving a shower:

- transfer from bed to shower commode chair

- move shower commode chair into bathroom

- shower

- dry and dress upper limbs

- move shower commode chair into bedroom

- transfer from shower commode chair to bed

- dress lower limbs in lying position

- transfer from bed to wheelchair.

Bringing it back to the example of the health professional who had to make a decision about a shower commode chair versus the bath shower trolley (discussed in chapter 9), the following table outlines the impact of implementing an activity analysis of each transfer option to make the decision. When compared against each other, we can see that the use of the shower commode chair results in three additional steps to the personal care routine. While a person with sitting balance is usually best suited to a shower commode chair rather than a bath shower trolley, the activity analysis outlined in the table highlighted that this was one of the exceptions to that traditional recommendation.

Shower commode chair	Bath shower trolley
1. Hoist transfer from wheelchair to bath shower trolley to undress*	1. Hoist transfer from wheelchair to bath shower trolley to undress
2. Wash the lower limb in lying (to avoid soiling the sling)**	2. Wash upper and lower body
3. Hoist transfer from bath shower trolley to shower commode chair	3. Dry upper and lower body
4. Wash upper and lower body	4. Dress upper body
5. Dry upper and lower body	5. Fit the pad
6. Dress upper body	6. Fit the lower limb clothing
7. Hoist transfer from shower commode chair to bath shower trolley	7. Hoist transfer from bath shower trolley to wheelchair
8. Fit the pad	
9. Fit the lower limb clothing	
10. Hoist transfer from bath shower trolley to wheelchair	

* Nearest bed to allow for undressing the lower limb was located on the opposite side of the house.

** The client would be significantly soiled when undressed and the shower commode chair did not provide sufficient access to wash the groin area efficiently.

How we do them: Objective assessment

During the assessment process, we also need to assess how well we are doing the activities involved in the manual handling process. In chapter 14 (principle 6), I provide more detail on how we can objectively assess a routine using regulation and policy, research, standardised testing or previously written safe work procedures.

Impact of environmental and personal factors

In chapter 1, I outlined the various personal and environmental factors that can influence the manual handling process. Using these headings, we can complete a check on those aspects of the person and the environment that are contributing positively and negatively to the manual handling process. While many of these may sound obvious, with more complex clients sometimes the manual handling routine may involve more than noticed at first glance. Using a framework such as the PEOP model allows the health professional to do a check to ensure all aspects of the person and the environment are considered in the assessment process.

In chapter 17 (principle 9) I discuss in more detail how these factors might influence manual handling – beyond a purely physical presentation – and how we might use this information to think of alternative solutions to manual handling problems.

Principle 5 summary

- Systematic assessment involves four steps: activity analysis, objective assessment, and analysis of personal and environmental factors.

- Activity analysis is the backbone of any manual handling risk assessment. Ensure you break down each mini step in the manual handling process as part of what you observe.

- Assess how we do manual handling routines with objective criteria in mind. This can include regulation and policy, research findings, objective assessments and safe work procedures. See chapter 14, principle 6, for further details.

- Both the personal and environmental factors can give us clues as to why a manual handling routine is as it currently stands. They can also provide guidelines on how we could strive to make a manual handling routine safer and more efficient. See chapter 17, principle 9, for more.

Activities

- How do you currently tackle manual handling assessments?

- How could you implement some of these guidelines to have a system for how you determine causes of challenges and how you look for solutions?

Principle 6: Implement objective guidelines

The balance between the needs of the care worker and the client is a challenging task in manual handling. The decisions we make to keep the care worker safe can have real consequences on the lives of people with disabilities. We need to know when we are making these decisions that they are based on something objective to guide our clinical reasoning. It is important to explain the objective criteria for a decision to our client and their care worker. And as health professionals, it is also important that we know the objective criteria behind our decisions so we can be confident in our clinical rationale, no matter how much we might want it to be a different conclusion. As outlined in the previous chapter, objectively looking at how we do manual transfers is an important part of the PEOP model, as is using it to assess for risk as well as opportunities for efficiencies.

In addition, Fisher and Ury talk about objective criteria from a negotiation standpoint. This direction towards objectivity enables us to take the emotion out of decisions that could otherwise be exceptionally emotional. When we balance this with the three other elements in the negotiation model (ensuring a win–win outcome, building a relationship and being efficient), we can support our client through these decisions – as opposed to mandating or 'playing the WHS card'.

Finding objective guidelines

A number of sources are available in practice to assist allied health professionals implement objective guidelines about 'how' we do manual handling. These include regulations and policy, research findings, standardised tests and safe work procedures.

Regulations and policy

Regulation and policy can form a boundary for what is and is not possible when assisting someone with a disability. These can then provide an objective reference point by which decisions are being made. For example, page 6 of the 2015 Australian Commonwealth Work Health and Safety (WHS) Code of Practice[1] states that a hazardous manual handling task is defined as 'a task that requires a person to lift, lower, push, pull, carry or otherwise move, hold or restrain any person'. A policy is the translation of this regulation into the workings of an organisation. In the care agency I used to work with, they would have extended this regulation to say a hazardous task required 'a caregiver to lift, lower, push, pull,

---

1   Workplace Health and Safety (2015). 'Hazardous Manual Tasks Code of Practice'. Made under the *Work Health and Safety Act 2011*, section 274. Retrieved 8 August 2017 from www.legislation.gov. au/Details/F2016L00406/Explanatory%20Statement/Text.

carry or otherwise move, hold or restrain any, all or most of the client's body weight unaided'. This was something objective I could use in practice to explain to the client what was possible in terms of how the care worker could assist them safely. As outlined in chapter 18 (principle 10), we discuss this objective measure with the client before my assessment of the task takes place.

Research

A strong research base in manual handling outlines what is safe and unsafe for a care worker. We can use this evidence to back up decisions we have to make and explain to stakeholders objectively as to why we are making these decisions specific to certain tasks. For example, Marras et al[2] found that it is not possible to lift someone of 50 kilograms safely without the likelihood of putting strain on the back, even when correct biomechanics are adhered to. This allows us to conclude that anyone who is supporting the majority of someone's weight, even if they are using 'correct biomechanics', is likely to sustain an injury.

In another example, a study by Fray and Hignett[3] compared a manual transfer to a mechanical aid in lying to sitting. They found 135 to 242N of strain on the back (depending on the size of the patient) by doing the transfer manually. With a mechanical aid, this was reduced to between 34 and 79N of strain on the back (depending on size of the patient). This helps us conclude that the first 30 degrees of the lying to sitting transfer is the most hazardous and mechanical aids can be effective at minimising this strain.

---

2   Marras, WS, Davis, KG, Kirking, BC, & Bertsche, PK. (1999). 'A comprehensive analysis of low-back disorder risk and spinal loading during the transferring and repositioning of patients using different techniques', *Ergonomics*, 42:7, 904–926, doi: 10.1080/001401399185207.

3   Fray, M, & Hignett, S. (2015). 'An evaluation of the biomechanical risks for a range of methods to raise a patient from supine lying to sitting in a hospital setting'. Paper presented at the 19th Triennial Congress of the IEA, Melbourne 9–14 August 2015.

Standardised testing

A number of standardised tests are also available that can help to quantify aspects of manual handling and 'how' we do them. When we are looking at ergonomic risk, a number of tools measure the deviation from the body in its neutral position. The body reaching a certain level of deviation from neutral can be a predictor of the likelihood of musculoskeletal injury (MSI) from manual handling. These include simple tools such as the rapid upper limb assessment (RULA)[4], rapid entire body assessment (REBA)[5] or the quick ergonomic check (QEC)[6].

These tools can provide a visual representation of risk for the client and care worker to help in understanding why a specific decision is made. We can use them as part of our assessment with a client or in evaluating the effectiveness of equipment, as outlined in chapter 16 (principle 8). While using these measures can be complex in practice, we can decide to use certain aspects or the idea of them to make them practical in a clinical setting. As a manual handling professional, I think it is important for us to know how these measures work regardless of whether we actually use them in practice.

Safe work procedures

Safe work procedures (SWPs) are another example of an objective measure, and their strength is that they are specific to a certain client. They are a representation of a procedure at a specific point in time and they outline the skills the client and the care worker

---

4   McAtamney L, Nigel Corlett, E. (1993). 'RULA: a survey method for the investigation of work-related upper limb disorders'. *Applied Ergonomics*, 24(2): 91–9.

5   Hignett S, McAtamney, L. (2000). 'Rapid entire body assessment (REBA)'. *Applied Ergonomics*, 31(2): 201–5.

6   'Quick Exposure Check (QEC)'. Retrieved 8 August 2017 from www.ergonomistswithoutborders.org/resources/downloads/QEC_Tool.pdf.

bring to the table to partner in the transfer process. With these documented, objectively seeing if a client's skill has deteriorated becomes less difficult, because you can identify when they are unable to bring the skills needed as outlined in the SWP. We can therefore quantify the 'gap' (as discussed in chapter 3), as opposed to it being something ambiguous.

For example, the safe work procedures could include '[Name] stands by the rail in the bathroom to allow the care worker to dress and undress the lower limbs'. If the client is no longer able to stand in the bathroom for this required period of time to allow the dressing of the lower limbs, then the client is clearly no longer in a position to function as is required in the SWP. The written SWP provides us with something around which to frame difficult conversations sensitively with a client.

Implementing objective guidelines in practice – the standing hoist

Implementing objective guidelines provides a way of framing reports on 'how' we are undertaking manual handling. Doing so takes the emotion out of the decisions we need to make and provides us with an argument for making decisions. Finding the balance in meeting the needs of both the client and the care worker is an essential component of any manual handling intervention – and hence the need for objective guidelines in making clinical decisions. An item of equipment that creates challenges in this regard is a standing hoist.

Standing hoists are a fantastic resource for the client and their caregiver. They allow the person to maintain independence and for both parties to significantly reduce the amount of steps in the transfer process. This means tasks such as toileting can be made a whole lot easier. However, while standing hoists are easy to prescribe, they are very hard to un-prescribe. They can also be recommended without sufficient guidelines for when they are safe to use – and when they become unsafe. These kinds of issues form a major theme in terms of questions I get from allied health professionals regarding standing hoists.

For a client and their caregiver, there is a significant change that occurs in a manual handling routine when moving from a standing hoist to a full lifting hoist. For the task of toileting alone, what was a two-step process when using the standing hoist becomes a four-step process when using the full lifting hoist. In terms of time use, the transition to a full lifting hoist impacts massively on care. This can result in both the client and the care worker continuing to use a standing hoist beyond the point at which it is safe.

As health professionals in manual handling, we need to be able to confidently advise on when a person needs to move from a standing hoist to a full lifting hoist. Given the massive implications this has for the client and their caregiver both practically and emotionally, we need to make sure this decision is the correct one.

Guidelines for the physical aspects

Our bottom line is to keep the care worker and their client safe. The word 'safe' can be very ambiguous because the word itself doesn't provide a tangible guide as to what is 'safe'. We need to have guidelines as to what safe looks like.

Looking through the existing literature, very few guidelines were provided for allied health professionals to determine what 'safe' in a standing hoist looks like. In fact, no research studies had addressed the use of a standing hoist. In 2016, my colleague Emma Small and I decided we needed to look at this[7]. We undertook a research study

---

7   Gallagher, A, & Small, E. (2016). 'Standing hoists: To stand or not to stand?' Paper presented at the Australian Association for the Manual Handling of People (AAMHP) Biennial Conference, Fremantle, Australia, 26 May 2016.

where we asked manual handling advisors what skills they felt clients needed to display for a standing hoist to be safe for both the care worker and the client. This study was the first step in drafting some guidelines for allied health professionals on the correct prescription of standing hoists. These guidelines can offer some kind of objective measure for health professionals in making the decision about whether someone is safe or unsafe in a standing hoist.

One outcome that came from this study was the importance of the lying to sitting transfer as part of the standing hoist assessment. This transfer can mean that at times a standing hoist can become unsafe for a care worker before it becomes unsafe for a client. Without the skills to be able to do the lying to sitting transfer with minimal assistance from the care worker or assistive technology, the standing hoist is something that becomes unsafe in terms of the care worker being able to assist. In addition, challenges can occur if the client lacks the skills to hold their torso upright when sitting on the side of the bed. The full results of this study will be published soon, and the pilot study can be found by visiting my website (www.riskmanaged.com.au).

In the prescription of a standing hoist, I recommend the introduction of an objective measure that illustrates safety. This document can be created from research findings such as those in our standing hoist study, and could outline the skills a client needs to display for the standing hoist to continue to be safe for the client and their care worker. The second part of this document could also outline what unsafe looks like and the key behaviours we would see the client doing, for the use of a standing hoist to be considered unsafe. Including pictures in this document of what unsafe and safe looks like can help the prescriber to be completely objective in the message sent. I recommend that both parties sign this document to outline their understanding of all objective measures.

Guidelines for the emotional aspects

Standing hoists promote a significant amount of independence and the decision on behalf of the allied health professional to disrupt that can be an emotionally charged process. It can challenge every philosophy that a health professional has been educated to believe in, and the health professionals can find themselves torn between safety for the care worker and client and the client's right to make a choice.

I get stories from health professionals all the time where they had a fantastic relationship with a client until it came to the point where they had to remove a standing hoist. Even years after this event, the relationship never recovered and care became a series of mini-conflicts where a trusting relationship was never re-established.

In the negotiation framework I introduced in chapter 9 (principle 1), Fisher and Ury discuss the importance of objective criteria. They discuss the psychology of decision-making where parties in a negotiation will want to see that decisions are being made in a fair and reasonable way. Even with tough decisions, once a person knows that a fair and reasonable process was used to arrive at a decision, they are less likely to have an objection to it.

A big aspect of removing a standing hoist from a client is miscommunication. While the health professional is removing the hoist for safety reasons for all parties, a client can sometimes misinterpret the decision as being based on the therapist being pro- or anti-rehabilitation and client autonomy. In some instances, clients can also misinterpret this action as 'personal'. In our intervention with our client, we need to ensure that this misinterpretation does not take place. This is where an objective measure can have a second use, because it outlines right from when the standing hoist is first prescribed the key behaviours that will indicate when it has become unsafe.

Timing in this process is critical. As outlined in the previous section, it is important to have this conversation about what unsafe looks like on supply of the standing hoist or, even better, during the intervention to first prescribe the standing hoist. This means mutual understanding is in place well before any issues arise – both the client and the care worker agree on the span at which standing hoists are appropriate for both parties. In the event the standing hoist becomes unsafe, the original prescribing document can be referred to as an objective measure as it explains why a decision is being made to remove the hoist. This not only gives the allied health professional confidence in making a clinical decision but also involves the client in the process and allows them to see, objectively, why this decision needs to be made.

Principle 6 summary

- Objective measures in practice enable us to take the emotional elements out of decisions that are exceptionally emotional.

- Regulations, policy, research findings, standardised measures and safe work procedures (SWP) are all examples of objective measures.

- Objective measures can be used to place guidelines on what safe and unsafe looks like with certain equipment – for example, a standing hoist.

- These objectives measures allow us to deal with the physical, social and emotional elements of a manual handling intervention as sensitively as we can.

Activities

- Think about which objective measure might be most applicable in your practice right now.

- How might you bring one of these objective measures into your practice to address the physical, social and emotional elements of your intervention?

Principle 7: Get creative

Our goal is to get the greatest utility from equipment at our disposal and take every available opportunity to eliminate manual handling. This can make the care of a person with a complex disability easier – for the person and their family, and for the care worker who supports them. When looking for hidden gems, we might find them in a technique or product, or in the ways we could use that product. In doing this, we also want to be able to leave the office with confidence that we have not compromised the bottom line of safety but we have unlocked some opportunities to make things easier. That is, we've moved beyond safety. Finding these opportunities often requires us to get a bit creative.

How can we use creativity?

Psychologist Mihaly Csikszentmihalyi is widely known for recognising and naming the psychological concept of flow, a highly focused mental state. In *Creativity: Flow and the psychology of discovery and invention*, he discusses creativity in terms of effective problem solving, where divergent ideas are used to find workable solutions. He links creativity with risk, identifying that to be creative is to take a risk[1].

How do we do this? By moving beyond the sole focus on safety, we need to start being creative. So, in the interventions we use and the equipment we prescribe, we need to know what creative use looks like.

Using our creativity is a funny one because, people either love it or they don't. I think people who get it, love it, and people who don't, hate it. People who hate creativity think it is a complete waste of time. Let's be clear here, however – the aim of creativity is to discover outcomes that work. It is about real, practical problem-solving and uncovering solutions you never knew were there. It is the process of trying things out, getting them spectacularly wrong, learning from this and then getting to a solution that is right.

A creative risk management model

You can use creative risk management as a vehicle to play and explore, and to help you to grasp all available opportunities to make manual handling routines as efficient as possible without losing sight of the bottom line of safety.

Creative risk management is a combination of creativity principles and risk management. The addition of creativity to the risk management process involves dividing the third step in the risk management process, which is risk control (as outlined in chapter 7), into two steps – that is, using divergent and convergent thinking. *Divergent* thinking involves identifying a number of options to control the problem. *Convergent* thinking involves testing these options using the usual risk control options to identify which are workable and which are not.

---

1 Csikszentmihalyi, M. (2013). *Creativity: Flow and the psychology of discovery and invention.* Harper Perennial.

So the three-part risk management process introduced in chapter 7 can be expanded creatively, as shown in the following figure.

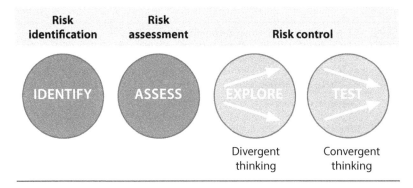

The model for creative risk management becomes as follows:

- *Risk identification:* First, we identify the problem to be solved or the process that could make a manual handling routine more efficient.

- *Risk assessment:* Next, we identify why it is a problem in its current state or why the current routine is cumbersome.

- *Explore:* Next, we get as creative as possible and explore options for alternative solutions.

- *Test:* Finally, we test all ideas. Does an idea work? Does it meet safety standards?

As shown in the preceding outline, this risk assessment process will always allow you to test each option to examine if it reaches the threshold of being safe before you ever bring a real client into the process. When it is not, the risk control process allows you to examine if these risky elements can be controlled and if this residual risk is acceptable. The table on the following page outlines the creative risk management model in more detail.

Creative risk management model

IDENTIFY

- Statement of the problem as you observed it or the process you would like to make better.

ASSESS

- Why is the current situation a problem?
- Is it something to do with the care worker or receiver?
- Is it something to do with the environment – physical, social, cultural?
- It is something to do with how the task is being done or the process of the task?
- What is the *likelihood* and *severity* of injury if things stay the same?

EXPLORE

Divergent thinking

What options are available? What would they look like?

For each option think about the following:

Positive implications:

- What problem might be solved if this action was put in place?
- Could any further opportunities or actions be made easier because of this?
- What is the likelihood of positive consequences?

Negative implications:

- Does a likelihood of any injury exist if this action was put in place?
- How might that occur?
- What would be the severity of the injury if an incident did take place?
- How can you enhance the positive/helpful actions and control the negative/unhelpful actions?

Rules:

- What rules are in place that you are required to follow?
- What rules apply and why?
- What rules are helping in this scenario?
- What rules are hindering in this scenario?
- What rules do not apply here and why?
- Can you justify going against an official rule?
- How can you prove that things will remain as safe as before but will be easier?

TEST

Convergent thinking

- With all the risky elements, how can you use the risk control hierarchy?
- Can you eliminate, substitute for a lesser one, isolate, introduce another item, or implement a guide or procedure?

Risk control hierarchy:

- eliminate
- substitute
- isolate
- use engineering controls
- use administrative controls.

Options to control risk:

- Describe all possible options.

Consider the residual risk

- Residual risk will always exist. Your aim here is to see if one item might have more residual risk than the other and why that is the case.
- Again, consider the *likelihood* and *severity* of injury as a result of residual risk.

Aims of creative risk management

The aim of creative risk management is to explore all possibilities. It can be used to:

- implement the fundamentals of the risk assessment process to explore options

- test out a rule to determine why it is there

- uncover new opportunities with equipment we already have in use

- identify the boundaries of what the available equipment can do

- check that every option passes the fundamentals of safety

- improve the training and continuing professional development environment so staff intimately know the equipment they use

- get the best out of the equipment in solving manual handling problems.

So creative risk management is a great tool to use for continuing professional development (CPD) events, allowing you to structure your learning. It can be used when equipment companies come to your workplace with new items of equipment. Instead of looking passively at the equipment or letting the representative lead the session, use the creative risk management process to take the lead, get in there, and explore. If you want to learn about equipment that you already use all the time, you can set up a learning event in your workplace to use creative risk management to identify all the possibilities of the equipment. Identify the problem you want to solve, and explore the equipment using the creative process to see what features on it (used in a variety of ways) could solve that problem.

You can then do the safety check at the end to see if the feature or process reaches the stage where it may be useful clinically with your clients. Instead of looking at things passively at conferences, get in there and start really looking at the equipment and testing it.

Think about some rules that have always bothered you. You can use creative risk management to test the rule against an alternative and see what happens.

We also need to know when we have crossed the line and we are entering the reckless area. An effective creative risk management model, as outlined in the following section, will help you do that. We can very easily be creative in our practice by thinking about the worst that could possibly happen and how we can control for that.

Implementing the model

The implementation of a model like this requires a significant gearshift in your thinking. Firstly, you need to be okay with asking silly questions and trying things out that are likely not to work. You need to be able to sometimes go against the thinking of people around you. This creative risk management model moves away from everything conservative and the rule-based mentality that you likely will have been used to in the manual handling space.

A big aspect of the principle of creativity is getting things wrong – which we, as adults, don't like. (Of course, children are excellent at being creative, and don't have any problem being wrong. For more on this, see the TED Talk 'Do schools kill creativity?' by Ken Robinson. In it, Robinson argues that children are born with innate creativity but they then have it educated it out of them!)[2]

Being wrong is also considered unprofessional so we aim to avoid it as much as possible. In manual handling in particular, we

---

2   www.ted.com/talks/ken_robinson_says_schools_kill_creativity?

have been told being wrong will lead to injury so anything that moves towards risk in any way is bad.

Try to get back to a state of childlike creativity and disregard for being wrong. Let's start to celebrate being wrong. Have fun with this, don't worry about being right, just explore and see what happens. Always test before you try anything to see if it is crossing the line into being unsafe before you ever bring a client into the mix. The aim of this process is not to go into the danger zone, but to stay within the range of safety with every procedure you use. Manual handling involves so many problems we are yet to solve. With our fundamental skills and development of creative problem-solving, we can create some innovative solutions to real problems.

Case study

To see the creative risk management model in action, let's look at an example of a rule I am asked about all the time: when transferring from a hoist to a chair, should brakes be used on the hoist or on the chair? Therapists ask me this question with a sense of embarrassment about even needing to ask it. It seems to relate to an area considered so basic that to ask about it surely indicates the therapist doesn't know what they're doing.

But this is a great question because therapists are often unsure of the answer. The question is often asked in the context of which is 'safer'. When we start examining the answer, however, we start to see this is not a safety question but an efficiency question.

In positioning from a hoist to a chair, with one care worker, what brakes go on where?

I am really interested in the process that happens when I ask this question. People rely on memory and what someone else has taught them when outlining what they do in practice. Instead of passively discussing it, health professionals need to get in there and work it out. The four combinations outlined in the following table are theoretically possible.

	Option 1	Option 2	Option 3	Option 4
Hoist brakes	On	Off	On	Off
Chair brakes	On	Off	Off	On

The following sections outline the findings if we use the creative risk management model to explore and test each of these options.

Option 1: Hoist and chair brakes on

Many mobile hoists lift in an arch, which means the distance between the chair and the hoist changes throughout the lift. With both brakes locked, the equipment does not allow for this distance change. The result is you have to make a really good guess of where the person is going to land on the chair before you position it. Because of the high probability of this guess being wrong, the care worker ends up doing a lot more manual handling to get the person positioned in the chair. If the chair and the hoist are too close, the client's head is likely to collide with the spreader bar of the hoist when they are lowered down into the chair.

Option 2: Hoist and chair brakes off

With both the hoist and chair brakes off, everything – all equipment – moves. Is this unsafe? Not necessarily – unless you have a really slippery floor on an incline so the hoist moves across the floor. It is, however, cumbersome because the care worker has to control two moving objects when positioning in the chair. They will use a lot more energy and will probably need two people involved. There is also the risk of the hoist boom colliding with the person when positioning in the chair.

Option 3: Hoist brakes on, chair brakes off

This option is where you can start to get some efficiency. Hoist brakes on and chair brakes off is a great option for positioning from the back. If you have a chair with mobile wheels, the care worker can position themselves at the back of the chair. Once the hoist gets the person to five centimetres above the seat of the chair, the care worker can pull them back into the seat of the chair, using their body to move the chair into position. With the hoist brakes locked, you get stability between the two items but you also get that slight mobility (in the chair) that is needed to deal with distance changes from the lifting arch.

Option 4: Hoist brakes off, chair brakes on

This option is good for positioning from the front. With the brakes on the wheelchair locked, the care worker can get leverage on the client's knees or hips to position the hips into the seat of the chair.

Based on the creative risk management exercise outlined here, I would recommend having both option 3 and 4 in your toolbox for positioning people into a seating position in their chair, dependent on whether you want to position from the back or the front. Remember – the Person–Environment–Occupation–Performance (PEO) model of occupational performance (outlined in chapter 1) gives you a checklist of things you need to consider when doing a full assessment of your client. Always do a check of the broader context in which care is provided to catch any factors that have the likelihood of tipping a practice into the hazardous range. (Also refer to chapters 13 and 14 (principles 5 and 6) for more on this.)

Principle 7 summary

- The aim of creative risk management is to explore all possibilities. It can be used to:
    - implement the fundamentals of the risk assessment process to explore options
    - test out a rule to determine why it is there
    - uncover new opportunities with equipment we already have in use
    - identify the boundaries of what the available equipment can do
    - check that every option passes the fundamentals of safety
    - improve the training and continuing professional development environment so staff intimately know the equipment they use.

- Creative risk management involves four steps: risk identification, risk assessment, convergent thinking and divergent thinking to control the manual handling risk.

- Creative risk management should only be used in continuing professional development (CPD) settings to safely explore equipment before ever introducing any concepts to a client situation.

Activities

Instead of trying to remember rules, test them out.

Get your local equipment supplier to bring the latest equipment options to you and use the creative risk management model to see how you can get the best out of each equipment item.

Think about equipment solutions you have at your disposal. How can you get to know what they can do better by using the creative risk management framework?

16

Principle 8: Use equipment evaluation to separate the gem from the gimmick

In the 1980s, a gap existed between manual handling requirements and equipment options available, because there was no real innovation in the industry. Carers of people with disabilities had to do a significant amount of lifting in providing assistance. As light was shed on the risk to carers from manual handling, especially the risk of back injury, industry experts put a call out for equipment innovators to develop solutions. By the start of the 21st century, these solutions were being provided by forward-thinking equipment companies. Innovators came to the industry, creating some really clever options to minimise manual handling. While they answered the call in terms of options available, we now have the opposite problem. We have too many options available to us.

The equipment innovation monster

We almost have it too good. Instead of one sling to lift someone from a chair, we now have 200; instead of one slide sheet, we now have 50 different types. Instead of solving a problem, allied health professionals started to become overwhelmed and anxious by the number of options available. Some participants of my workshops have continuously described the feeling of dread when presented with 20 sling options, and of not really knowing where to even start. They describe feeling vulnerable when talking to an equipment representative and being reliant on the equipment representative to tell them which piece of equipment they need, as opposed to being able to make that decision clinically themselves. Workshop participants told me that they were often fearful they would be sold a useless gimmick if they deviated from the norm and so were more likely to go with what they knew.

The second problem was that sometimes allied health professionals didn't have the skills to be able to use the equipment available to them. They never really got a chance to play around with it, get comfortable with it and feel confident with it. They never felt they reached a level of confidence to be able to competently show it to a client who was sometimes unwell or was struggling with the transition to needing help.

In the workshops I run and the conferences I present at, I am exposed to vast amounts of equipment. Therapists explain to me that they are overwhelmed by the amount of choice available when they go to these events. Some allied health professionals go to conferences and see new equipment but they don't know how to engage with it. They don't know how to check it out, play with it and learn about it so they can see what it would be like in practice. Sometimes we need to compare equipment to something else to really see its value. This comparison is key in the decision-making process for therapists.

This situation has led to a vicious cycle of therapists feeling overwhelmed by choice and so sticking with what they know. This has meant that some amazing equipment solutions have been left on the shelf because they were identified as a gimmick when they are really a gem. In saying that, some equipment solutions are gimmicks and we need to avoid them. Allied health professionals need to have the skills to be able to differentiate one from the other.

The challenge for the innovator

I think historically a disconnect has existed between allied health professionals and equipment providers. Equipment providers traditionally come from a sales background and so making a sale has been the outcome of success. I have talked to many equipment companies as I've researched the new items available for manual handling over the last number of years. While a sales representative is in a sales role, many I have spoken ultimately want to solve a problem. If their product doesn't solve a problem, they don't want to sell it.

The shortfall of research

Research has guided the science of manual handling, and we are fortunate that a lot of research is available that outlines what works to reduce injury. Unfortunately, research is also very good at telling us what does not work. This can make decision-making really challenging because in practice we can't do nothing; we need to come up with a solution to the problem.

One of the challenging responses I get from people I mentor on evidence-based practice is that academic journals never mention their specific situation. Allied health professionals find it difficult to transfer the knowledge from the research to the situation that is in front of them clinically. Research has many standards to pass before it can be deemed conclusive research, resulting in sometimes long and complicated methods. This makes it hard for health professionals to see what this might have to do with their practice. What research papers do have, however, is a methods section that shows how objective decisions were made from this research perspective. These methods can be an excellent clinical reasoning tool in justifying decisions in practice.

I had the pleasure of listening to Dr Susan Gallagher speak at a recent seminar at Concord Hospital Sydney. During her talk I asked her how we are doing in equipment innovation in terms of the care of the person of size[1]. Echoing my own thoughts on manual handling equipment available generally, Dr Gallagher said she felt we had all the equipment innovations we needed – they were just not being used as well as they could be. She felt that if any more than four members of staff were at any bedside in the manual handling of a person of size, the wrong equipment was being used.

Four steps to assessing and exploring equipment

As allied health professionals we need to become proficient at evaluating equipment. We need to use our time at conferences, where we initially see new equipment, to assess it and differentiate the gimmick from the gem. We need to be able to do that first screening process in our heads so that we can more efficiently target what equipment solution might solve a certain manual handling problem.

---

1 Gallagher, S. (2017). 'The needs of a person living with obesity'. Paper presented at the Bariatric Management Innovation Seminar Series, Concord Hospital, Sydney, Australia, 8 February 2017.

In my moving and handling programs and workshops, I introduce the four steps shown below to help explore equipment.

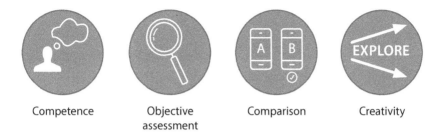

| Competence | Objective assessment | Comparison | Creativity |

Remember – in using this model, we need to keep our investigation to one singular manual handling activity. Some of these activities can include:

- rolling on a bed
- lifting legs to attend to personal care
- fitting a hoist sling in lying
- fitting a hoist sling in sitting
- positioning in a wheelchair using a hoist
- positioning in a wheelchair without a hoist
- lying to sitting transfer
- sitting to lying transfer
- sit to stand transfer
- stand to sit transfer
- stand pivot transfer
- transfer off the floor
- sliding transfer from chair to chair

- transfer into a car from standing
- transfer into a car from sitting.

Competence

Before we use equipment, we need the skill set to know how to use it. This may mean asking the equipment representative to demonstrate how the item works so you know the steps to get the best out of the item. Coupled with this, the allied health professional may need to up skill themselves on the basics of safe manual handling. With the allied health professional acting as the caregiver, this may involve examining the extent to which they find themselves deviating from neutral spine – not because the procedure demands it but because of the way they are positioning their body. With the allied health professional acting as the caregiver, this can be as much about habit and awareness as it is about skills. While we may be great at telling others about the extent to which they are deviating from neutral spine, we might find our own practice is poor. (I have indeed been guilty of that.)

Objective assessment

Objective assessment helps allied health professionals move away from the 'I like/I don't like' subjective analysis of equipment. It helps to pinpoint why and in what context an item of equipment is of value. We do this by applying assessments (based on objective criteria used in research) to regular clinical cases that would be present in practice. These skills form the basis of a comprehensive assessment that could be used in practice to clinically justify equipment.

This is the 'bottom line' stuff. Ask yourself what really matters in the care of this person with a disability, and for their family and the care worker who assists them. As a therapist, what is the measure of a good outcome for this person? You can then assess and collect data based on this measure.

The data we collect can be either numbers-focused or words-focused – that is, it can be quantitative or qualitative. While qualitative research has increased in its value, numbers still rule with decision-makers, whether we like it or not.

We need to play the numbers game in our practice. The good news is that some simple tools are available to help us do this and so justify our cause and get some great outcomes for our clients with physical disabilities and the people who care for them.

Some data you could collect includes:

- number of steps in the process

- cost of installed items (including maintenance costs)

- level of deviation from neutral position of body/ergonomic risk

- experience and comfort (for client and care worker)

- time taken to complete the procedure

- number of care workers required

- cost of the procedure

- time for the item to pay for itself.

Number of steps in the process
The first step in the assessment of any manual handling routine is to complete an activity analysis (chapter 13, principle 5). Accounting for each step of the process can give us an indication of the level of complexity within a procedure. This in turn can provide a good reference point when performing an initial comparison of options.

Level of deviation from neutral spine

In manual handling, we are trying to minimise strain on the care worker. A measure of the exposure to manual handling that can cause musculoskeletal injury is the extent to which the body deviates from neutral, beyond what is considered within the safe limits of the body. Postures that place care workers at risk can include bending, twisting and overreaching. Formal tools measure this deviation from neutral spine when undertaking activities, including the rapid upper limb assessment (RULA)[2], the rapid entire body assessment (REBA)[3] or the quick exposure check (QEC)[4].

The score generated through an assessment such as one of these enables comparison between two different products or procedures. Even if you decide not to use something formal, the concept of measuring the extent and time spent deviating from neutral body position can be a useful comparison. We are not looking to do formal research here, just apply some principles for making objective assessments.

Experience and comfort

Measuring comfort and the experience of using a product or procedure is important. It needs to be a positive experience for everyone. You can collect data in this area qualitatively or quantitatively. If you ask people for their experience when using a certain piece of equipment, for example, they will give an answer, and you can include these responses in your data. You can also ask people to rate their experience on a scale. While you won't get complete reliability and validity in a scale, you are getting some kind of quantitative measure that will be a lot stronger in a report.

---

2   McAtamney L, Nigel Corlett E. (1993). 'RULA: a survey method for the investigation of work-related upper limb disorders'. *Appl Ergon*, 24(2): 91–9.

3   Hignett S, McAtamney L. (2000) 'Rapid entire body assessment (REBA)'. *Appl Ergon*, 31(2): 201–5.

4   'Quick Exposure Checklist'. Retrieved 8 August 2017 from www.ergonomistswithoutborders.org/resources/downloads/QEC_Tool.pdf.

Time for the procedure

The timing of a procedure is a critical measure because it gives an indication of the cost of a care worker providing that care. It could be assumed that the shorter the time required, the cheaper the care. This has benefits not only in terms of cost, but also in terms of quality of life for the client. With manual handling being the bridge to life, the less time the client needs to spend on that bridge, the more time the client gets to participate in the things that really matter to them. (We need to balance this, of course, with not compromising safety.)

Number of care workers

We need to examine the minimum number of care workers needed for care to be safe. Achieving a safe routine with one person can result in massive savings in terms of care costs. Many items of equipment can reduce the number of care workers needed in providing care from two to one, and sometimes three to one. Our assessment here is to check that safety is maintained if care by one care worker is achieved with the correct use of equipment. (Refer to chapter 11 (principle 3), where I talk about the benefits of care being managed by one person and how this can keep the cost of care down.) If two care workers are needed, not only do we need to double the cost of care but there might also be other additional costs in terms of the administration of the care.

Total cost of the procedure

Cost always comes into care, whether we like it or not. It can be useful to calculate the total cost of the procedure, comparing equipment to no equipment and in terms of the day-to-day delivery of that care. We can then calculate the cost of care per week, month or even per year.

Time taken for the item to pay for itself

By dividing the cost of the equipment by the difference between the daily cost of care with and without the item, you can calculate the number of days it would take for the item to pay for itself. It is also important to factor in any maintenance cost of the equipment. The following table shows an example of these workings.

	With item	Without item
Cost of care per day	$40 (a)	$80 (b)
Cost of care only per year (249 working days)	$9960	$19,920
Cost of item (including maintenance costs)	$5000 (c)	$0
Total cost of care per year	$14,950	$19,920
Number of days for item to pay for itself $5000/($80 – $40) (c) / (b) – (a)	125 days	

A real challenge here, however, is that the funder of the equipment and the beneficiary of the equipment in terms of money saved may not necessarily be the same person or entity. For example, an equipment pool may have a role to ensure a client is safe. They don't really have a priority to reduce the cost of care because this cost does not come out of their budget. This is a challenge for allied health professionals in justifying equipment.

While the dollar value does have merit, remember that is not the only factor that would justify a procedure. An item could offer no cost savings or impact on the safety of the care workers but may make for a more efficient experience in the care process of all parties. This is why all measures need to be taken into consideration when making objective decisions.

Comparison

Comparing is critical, because this allows you to see the benefit of one solution by comparing it to the alternative. This is explained in detail in chapter 12 (principle 4). It can be useful to compare the new product to what you know and also to no product, because considering equipment in isolation can make it difficult to come to any conclusions. This means you run through the same objective assessment points for each comparison.

We compare the quality of the item, servicing offered by the company and total cost of the item to complete a comprehensive cost benefit analysis of equipment.

The following table outlines how you could record your comparisons.

Activity	No equipment	Item 1	Item 2	Item 3
Number of steps				
Cost of installed item				
Deviation from neutral body/ ergonomic risk				
Experience and comfort (client)				
Experience and comfort (care worker)				
Time taken to complete the procedure				
Number of care workers				
Total cost of the procedure (time × hourly cost of care), per day/week/month/year				
Time for the item to pay for itself (cost of item ÷ difference between daily cost of care with and without item)				
Servicing/after-purchase care				

Creative risk management

Once you know what the equipment can do for your client in the traditional sense, the next stage is to start being creative. We take all the equipment we look at through the creative risk management process to see if any hidden gems are contained within the equipment in terms of its application. While always having safety as the bottom line, creative risk management can really help you get double bang for your buck out of all the equipment you use. As discussed previously, this is a process solely for exploration in the office environment or training space with colleagues, where rigorous testing of the idea takes place. It is not first introduced in the client's home.

Principle 8 summary

- Equipment innovators are coming up with creative solutions to solve manual handling problems.

- As allied health professionals, we need to be able to use objective criteria by which to differentiate the gimmick from the gem.

- Key measures include deviation from neutral spine, number of care workers required, time taken to complete the routine, care worker report, client report, cost of care and cost of the item.

- Comparisons allow you to see what the solution in question looks like when compared to the next best alternative.

- Once you know an item of equipment is of use, explore how you can get the best use out of the item using creative risk management.

Activities

- Think about inviting equipment representatives to your workplace to demonstrate new equipment solutions.

- Create a list of the objective criteria you are going to use to assess the item.

- Get your team to rate the item under these measures, comparing it to the scores you would get with the methods or equipment you already use.

Principle 9: Consider alternatives to get an outcome

The process of manual handling involves the physical moving of someone from one space to another with the assistance of a caregiver. It involves the client bringing skills and the caregiver partnering with them to help them fill in the gaps in function to get an outcome.

Manual handling is labelled a 'physical intervention' and traditionally it is. That is, if you see a physical problem in manual handling (that is, someone's inability to move themselves), you intervene by providing physical assistance. When factors such as cognitive impairment, intellectual disability or challenging behaviours enter the picture, this can become more difficult. While someone may have the physical capacity and fitness to do something, barriers may exist to them participating. In addition, some clients can be inconsistent in the extent to which they can participate or may indeed work against the functional task.

The care worker is expected to achieve a particular outcome – that is, that the person's personal care is attended to, including showering, toileting and dressing, if they are unable to do it themselves. In a morning routine, in a group home setting for example, the outcome may be that the person is sitting in the van ready for a day program or whatever daily activity they are engaged in. This may be in the context of assisting other clients with the added time pressure of ensuring this is done in an efficient fashion. Regardless of these added pressures, the expectation still exists that these functional self-care tasks are attended to and this involves manual handling.

The challenges with intervening physically

When a person is unable to participate in a task, we can intervene physically to assist them with what is a physical task. This is only appropriate, however, if the only barrier to them participating is physical – that is, their muscles won't work to get them from a to b and so we intervene to make up for that physical deficit. If an additional reason exists, beyond a physical one, which is affecting their ability to take part in the task, we enter a status where we complete the task without addressing the barrier to them participating. Using strategies like this we can find ourselves implementing what would be considered to have elements of restrictive practice. According to the Australian Law Reform Commission, 'Restrictive practices involve the use of interventions and practices that have the effect of restricting the rights or freedom of movement of a person with disability'[1]. Our aim is to achieve a safe and efficient transfer and the least restrictive alternative. When we talk about safety, we are not just talking about physical safety but safety from a mental standpoint also. Behaviourists would argue a reason always exists behind

---

1   Australian Law Reform Commission. (2017) *Restrictive Practices in Australia*. Retrieved 8 August 2017 from www.alrc.gov.au/publications/8-restrictive-practices/restrictive-practices-australia.

a person's behaviour. As allied health professionals, we need to be able to uncover the 'whys' behind this behaviour and so identify some strategies to address these barriers.

Understanding the why

The PEOP model introduced in chapter 1 (and shown again below) outlines the factors that come into play in manual handling. As already discussed, these factors include intrinsic or personal factors and extrinsic or environmental factors that influence the success of achieving a safe and efficient transfer for all parties. Using a model like this, we can start to understand some of the reasons a task such as toileting or showering, or ultimately achieving the outcome of assisting a client to sit in the van ready for a day program might be challenging. Understanding the why allows us to use that why to determine ways of addressing these barriers. If we get the why wrong, we can cause a significant amount of stress for the client and the care worker who supports them.

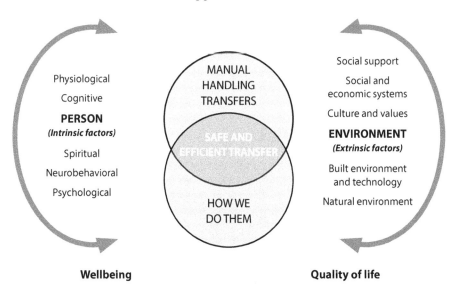

Physiological

Cognitive

PERSON
(Intrinsic factors)

Spiritual

Neurobehavioral

Psychological

MANUAL HANDLING TRANSFERS

SAFE AND EFFICIENT TRANSFER

HOW WE DO THEM

Social support

Social and economic systems

Culture and values

ENVIRONMENT
(Extrinsic factors)

Built environment and technology

Natural environment

Wellbeing   **Quality of life**

Personal (intrinsic factors)

If a safe and efficient transfer cannot be achieved it could be because of the following personal 'whys':

- *Physiological:* Even though they have the physical skills, they don't have the strength and endurance to be able to do the transfer.

- *Cognitive:* They are not able to understand what is being asked of them, recall the task they are being asked to do or have the attention needed to participate in the task fully.

- *Spiritual:* This task may not have any meaning for them.

- *Neurobehavioural:* They may not have the motor capacity to complete the task, or the neural pathways are impaired. In addition, sensory barriers may be present, in that they are unable to process something in the environment they are seeing, hearing, smelling, feeling or tasting. Pain could be a factor for them. Touch can also have an impact – are our hands hot or cold, rough or soft, for example? Tone of voice is also important – how does this impact on the client's behaviour?

- *Psychological:* They may be anxious or fearful about what they are being asked to do and not feel they have the skills to do it effectively.

Environmental (extrinsic factors)

A safe and efficient transfer may not be achievable because of the following environmental factors:

- *Social support:* The emotional, information and practical support being offered may be inadequate for staff or client.

- *Social and economic systems:* The political drive or economic means to provide support may not be present.

- *Culture and values:* A mismatch may exist between the culture and values of the care centre providing care and that which promotes a safe and efficient transfer regime. Does a difference exist between the formal and informal culture of the organisation? What policy does the centre work under? Similarly, the client's culture and values may be at odds with the workings of the centre or service providing care. Are they from a different cultural background?

- *Built environment and technology:* The physical environment and the equipment within it may not support a safe and efficient transfer regime.

- *Natural environment:* The outside environment may have barriers for the client in accessing the assistance of staff.

Understanding the why is critical to being able to address the barriers to the safe and efficient transfer. Uncovering this why can require quite a lot of observing as well as consulting with experts on the healthcare team. Expertise accessed can include behavioural psychologists, occupational therapists with skills in sensory and behavioural interventions as well as physiotherapists. These experts, in consultation with management, can help you uncover some of the intrinsic barriers and extrinsic factors at play, and so help achieve the safe and efficient outcome.

The Implementation of alternatives: The client with anxiety

I recently assessed a client who was very anxious about personal care routines. He had a developmental delay so it was difficult to offer reassurance to him verbally and ease his anxiety. We got the sense he found the care routines really anxiety-provoking, even though care was as gentle as possible. This was a real challenge for the care worker addressing his needs and resulted in a significant manual handling problem.

We could solve this problem by introducing another person to ease the manual handling burden. But what if we were to look at it another way and see if we could instead reduce the anxiety (the *psychological barrier*) that was causing the physical problem?

You can use two methods to help someone become less anxious. The first option is to talk to them about it. This is usually in the category of cognitive behavioural therapy (CBT), and involves reasoning with the person, who can then engage with you on a conversational level. You can use facts and reasoned conversation to help ease their anxiety. You can say, for example, 'It seems to me you feel really anxious at the moment. Tell me about that … What do you think would help us help you?' and so on.

With a client like the one I mentioned above, reasoning was not possible because he didn't have the cognitive skills to do that. So we needed to use another option. Trying to engage on a conversational level can be the default option but it can very often be ineffective with people with developmental delay who are unable to comprehend what is being said (a *cognitive barrier*) unless the care worker has a really strong relationship with the client.

The second option is to try to change the behaviour without the cognitive bit. This is where you distract. In this example, if we could focus the client's attention on something else other than the personal care, we could change their behaviour so they were a calmer, less rigid client. This client loved music so the care workers put on his favourite music during personal tasks. His anxiety reduced significantly because he was encouraged to focus on something he liked. This meant he was less resistant during personal care tasks and the manual handling was reduced. In addition, a very skilled care worker talked to him about something he was going to do in his day that he was looking forward to. This also distracted him from an activity that needed to happen as part of his overall care. For the client, their personal care routine – which they have to endure every day – was a little more pleasant an experience.

The falling client

Take the hypothetical example of a client with an intellectual disability who had the ability to walk. At a group home and during the day program, he lowers himself to the ground, sits and refuses to get up even though he had the physical capabilities to do so. The group home requests a hoist to be able to transfer this client off the ground.

We need to investigate two opportunities before we explore physical interventions in this case. Firstly, we need to understand why this client is displaying the behaviour of dropping to the floor. An antecedent is present here – that is, a sign or thing that happened before the behaviour. By studying his behaviour in these situations, we can draw some conclusions as to why he is making the decision to sit onto the ground.

From an intrinsic (personal) perspective some theories could be:

- *Physiological:* He doesn't have the strength or endurance to stay in standing.

- *Cognitive:* He is interpreting cues from his environment incorrectly to sit on the ground.

- *Spiritual:* Sitting on the ground has meaning for him.

- *Neurobehavioural:* From a motor perspective, he may not be able to stand or, from a sensory perspective, he is over- or under-stimulated by his environment.

- *Psychological:* He is emotionally unable to continue with the task of walking.

We can then intervene at that level to distract him from sitting and lead him towards more productive behaviour.

The second opportunity is examining what sitting on the ground means for him and his environment (both staff and other clients). Is his sitting on the ground a problem and, if so, why? Is the location where he is choosing to sit the problem more than the act of sitting? For example, is he sitting in a key passageway? If it is a problem in terms of the overall workings of the group home, we may need to find opportunities where he can display this behaviour in a more suitable environment.

Finally, to assist the client up from the ground, we need to give the client the opportunity to do this independently from a physical perspective. Do any physical barriers exist and how can we eliminate these? Does he just need time to process the task? We may also be able to change the sensory environment to support his behaviour. Does he like to do something that would provide the motivation to get up? A behavioural psychologist can be a significant resource in situations like this to find alternative psychological solutions to manual handling interventions.

What if the client does not assist?

At times a client has the physical capabilities to do a functional task, yet is unable to complete it on demand for cognitive, psychological, spiritual, neuro-behavioural or physiological reasons, even when the alternative interventions are put in place. This is a challenging situation, especially when the tasks the care workers are required to complete have a time component on them, and they do not have the allocation of additional resources to wait for a client to independently undertake the tasks. Without the luxury of time, the client's function becomes dysfunctional.

In situations like this, we may need a rehabilitation plan to facilitate learning of the tasks to get them to a functional level. We need to be careful, however, not to make these tasks 'the rehabilitation', with the expectation that a client can practice and relearn during functional tasks.

Instead, this may mean intense health professional intervention that is rehabilitative in nature, to enable the client to reach the skills both physically, cognitively and emotionally to participate meaningfully. In turn, this may mean added resources that allow for the contingencies when the client is unable to participate in the task. A client needs to be able to display base-level specific skills consistently with appropriate health professional intervention for these to really work in a day-to-day setting where self-care is the functional task.

Principle 9 summary

- Manual handling problems don't always need a 'physically' focused intervention to solve them.

- A safe and efficient outcome is from a mental health and wellbeing perspective as well as a physical one.

- Non-physical barriers may exist to a person participating in a task and, as allied health professionals, we need to identify the non-physical barriers to manual handling. Models such as the PEOP can provide us with a framework to start understanding 'the why'.

- Once the non-physical barriers are identified, we need to address them to achieve the outcome of a safe and efficient transfer.

- We need to work in collaboration with other health professionals such as behavioural psychologists, occupational therapists with skills in sensory processing, and physiotherapists. We also need to work with management to understand the broader environmental implications that could affect the client's care as well as the care worker supporting them.

Activities

- Do you have clients on your case load where manual handling is a problem yet the root of the problem is non-physical?

- Use the PEOP model to explore the 'why' behind the problem, and to explore what intervention might address the barriers to participation in the manual handling task.

- Can you change something in the environment that could ease manual handling? For example:
  - Is the visual environment too stimulating for the client?
  - Is the visual environment not stimulating enough?
  - Is the environment full of the wrong noise?
  - Could you distract and soothe the client with a certain kind of music or noise?

- How are you or care workers touching the client? Are hands warm or cold? Are you warning the client before you do something, or telling them what you are doing? Are you using their name to get attention?

- Are you giving clear directions?

Principle 10: Use the assessment guide

The PEOP model introduced in chapter 1 highlights that manual handling is a 'we' activity. It involves the partnership between a client and a care worker who supports them. By virtue of the fact that it is a 'we' activity, we cannot assess manual handling in isolation, and trying to do so is the biggest problem I feel we currently have in manual handling. A health professional working with the client may assess rehabilitation in isolation and a health professional working with the care worker may assess them in isolation. But both parties come to the table to participate in one activity, together.

Manual handling is a physical, social and emotional activity. In the assessment process, we need to be able to manage these elements. Without this focus, we can experience 'assessment creep' where the assessment process goes on long beyond the time of the face-to-face assessment due to the needs of the various stakeholders involved. This home visit assessment guide is designed to allow the health professional to manage these physical, social and emotional elements in the most time-efficient way possible, while implementing the principles related to assessment in the book.

The home visit initial assessment guide

This home visit assessment guide brings together the principles in the book that relate to how an assessment would take place in the home in relation to manual handling. I recommend that any assessment in the home should involve the client, family and the care worker being present. This assessment process has five main steps, which I go through in the following sections. These steps assume that the health professional has developed a therapeutic relationship with the client, family and care worker.

As advocated in chapter 9, I always suggest seeing the transfers in the real scenario as opposed to the dry run. This allows the assessor to address the real issues – which are sometimes not fully appreciated in the dry run.

Step 1: Ensuring all team members are present when manual handling is discussed

As manual handling is a 'we' activity, all team members must be present when manual handling is the focus. This sends the message that the needs of both parties are equally important in the manual handling process. This can be really challenging when multiple care agencies are involved as well as family. So, in all manual handling assessments, I 'invite' all members to the assessment. This highlights the importance of their perspective and the equal importance of the needs of all parties.

Getting agencies to buy into this concept can be a difficult process, and one that doesn't happen overnight. When encouraging anyone to come to the table on these things, you have to make it worth their while. As a business mentor of mine once said, keep it 'about them, about them, about them'. As allied health professionals, we have to sell the idea of care agencies turning up to this assessment. We need to show what they can gain out of it in terms of cost and time savings. We need to get their managers on board through helping them understand that coming to this manual handling assessment is in their best interests and they are missing out on tips to avoid injury, to make the job easier and to conserve their energy if they don't attend. You can learn lots from the available literature on negotiation and persuasion when working out how to get agencies to buy into this. (While outside the focus of this book, I am looking forward to writing my second book on negotiation.)

It is important to note that only a key representative from the care agency – perhaps the key care worker – needs to be present for the assessment, as opposed to the whole team. Even with this, if more than one agency is involved, a large number of people may still be present. This can be overwhelming for the client, considering a very intimate part of their lives is the focus of the assessment. The health professional needs to manage these to ensure only the parties who really need to be present, are present, to observe the intimate parts of the assessment. The assessor also needs to ensure the client has control of this and is aware of who will be present before the assessment commences. This might involve discussing this with the client privately first, to determine what parts they wish to have complete privacy during the assessment and how they can feel confident it is a dignified process for them.

Step 2: Provide a pre-assessment brief before viewing what is happening

This pre-assessment brief has five aims:

1 *Set time frames for the assessment:* You may have 1.5 hours for the assessment, so you need to outline what you need to get done in that time. Once people have a time limit in place, they are much more focused on getting to what the outcome is quicker.

2 *Highlight why you are there:* You need to sell to all parties that you are there to make things easier for them. Your role is to come up with a transfer routine where care is efficient and effective so the care worker is safe and the client feels confident and in control. You can make the transfers as fluid as possible, so they both can get on with all the other activities of daily living.

3 *Determine the issues:* Before starting an assessment, I always try to have a discussion with all parties present on what the issues are (refer to chapter 9, principle 1). I like to hear from the client, the family and the care worker. My role in this process is to summarise the issues and recode them from 'people' to 'problem'. I can then be soft on the people but tough on the problem. The 'manual handling transfers' are the problem, not the people behind them. It is here that you might need to address grief with the client, as outlined in chapter 10 (principle 2). Giving this discussion adequate but structured time is really important.

4 *Introduce an objective measure to the assessment:* As discussed in chapter 14, principle 6, people always want to know that the results of an assessment are fair and reasonable, and

we achieve this by setting an objective measure. If we can demonstrate that the objective measure has or has not been met, then people are less likely to have a problem with the outcome of the assessment. The objective measure needs to be disclosed to all stakeholders before the assessment starts as opposed to when there is a problem. At this stage, the health professional can be clear about what assessment tool they use to make decisions on what they see. This is where you can discuss the policy you work under and the boundaries of what you can work with. It is really important to talk about policies as an opportunity to offer some guidance, as opposed to something heavy and legislative. Once you have the boundaries of what is possible and not possible from the policy, you can be creative when working within that.

5   *Set ground rules in terms of discussing the assessment:* A pre-assessment discussion is an opportunity to establish some ground rules for how people are to behave during the assessment. At one extreme end, these rules allow you to deal with any challenging personalities. Having some group rules agreed to by all parties means you can refer to them if things get out of hand. It also allows you to introduce the idea of exploring options. Think about framing it in how you want people to behave as opposed to lecturing people on 'bad behaviour'.

Step 3: Observe and ask questions

Your role here is to observe the current routine and complete an activity analysis of what you see and objectively assess the various steps (refer to chapter 13, principle 5). Try to say as little as possible but let the parties involved share their experiences during this process. You don't need to give any solutions at this stage. Praise any good teamwork, communication or work practices you see. Speak for the client if they can't speak and you feel things could be better – for example, '[Name], I get the sense you might like to be covered up doing this procedure'. Use this as a time to continue to build a relationship with the team you are working with. Listen to any suggestions people have without judgement. Only intervene at this stage if you see something that crosses the line into being unsafe.

Step 4: Post-assessment brief

At this stage, you can revisit the goals of the assessment in achieving a safe and efficient, energy-saving transfer routine and you can have a chat about what you saw. Each person has the opportunity to have their say (refer to chapters 9 and 10 (principles 1 and 2)). It is at this time that you can compare what you saw, to the objective measures you've already outlined as a means of assessing the transfer routine (refer to chapter 14 (principle 6)). This is where the things that are going well are accounted for and the things that are going outside the declared objective measure can be identified.

For the aspects that are considered unsafe, together you then can ask the question, what do we do about it? Each member of the team gets to give their opinion. Allow people to be creative about it. At this stage, try to separate the process of coming up with options from the process of assessing them. Write all options down.

Because you have the objective measures set for the boundaries on what can and can't happen, you can introduce the idea of putting your team thinking hats on to come to a resolution together. Everyone involved works with you to come up with an answer, rather than you as the health professional providing the answer.

Step 5: Come up with an action plan

Your final stage is to come up with an action plan. This involves examining each of the ideas created in the post-assessment briefing and checking them off against the policy that you are working under. Completing this process can eliminate many options that are beyond the scope of what is safe. Checking them off the already established 'objective measure' means the objective measure, not you the health professional, is making the decision.

The final step is to clarify, where to from here? What do you want to trial to solve this problem? Here you can also come up with a strategy for the ongoing intervention in this outcome.

At this stage, it can be a good idea to do a check with the client privately to see how they are feeling about the assessment process and ask if they have any further questions about the process (refer to chapter 9 (principle 1)).

Dealing with the time factor

Allied Health Professionals consistently suggest to me that they don't have the time to have a meeting before and after an assessment visit. However, these visits need not take an excessive amount of time if you set time frames before you start. This can be as short as ten minutes before and after the assessment. If things go off track, you can refer back to the timing agreement and then get all team members back on track. Our aim is to complete an assessment in the most effective and efficient way possible.

Principle 10 summary

In assessing manual handling routines, a strategy to manage the physical, social and emotional elements is necessary. This enables the assessor to address these elements in the most effective and efficient way possible.

The assessment guide involves five steps:

1 Ensuring all team members are present when manual handling is discussed

2 Providing a pre-assessment brief before viewing what is happening

3 Observing and asking questions

4 Preparing a post-assessment brief

5 Coming up with an action plan

Activities

Give yourself a score out of ten for the following (with 1 being terrible and 10 being remarkable). How effective are you at:

– planning your assessments that involve manual handling

– addressing the physical elements

– addressing the social elements

– addressing the emotional elements.

Rank your scores from best to worst.

Think about what you can do to increase your score by 10 per cent in the three worst scoring areas.

Conclusion

In contemporary practice, the management of manual handling risk can be a complicated process. While meeting the needs of the client, we also need to manage the needs of the care workers. Their job is only getting more challenging due to the complex needs now presenting in the community. These caregivers have the right to return home to their families injury free.

In *The Manual Handling Revolution*, I have outlined a method where we as allied health professionals can manage the needs of all parties. To do this we need to:

- understand it's a negotiation, and prepare a strategy for managing the needs of all parties

- address the grief, and support the client in the process of change that may happen as a result of the assessment

- stop throwing care workers at the problem, and identify when a manual handling routine can be safely done by one care worker

- manage the manual handling neurosis, and close a case with the confidence we have done the best we can at eliminating manual handling risk

- use systematic assessment, and be confident that we are addressing every aspect at play in the assessment process

- implement objective guidelines, and be transparent in where our decisions come from

- get creative, and unlock all the opportunities to eliminate manual handling hidden in an innovative product, and use these safely

- use equipment evaluation to separate the gem from the gimmick, and learn about new equipment and opportunities to eliminate manual handling and better the lives of people with disabilities and the care workers who support them

- consider alternatives to get an outcome, and expand our toolbox for solving manual handling problems beyond just physical interventions

- use the assessment guide, and practically implement all these principles in a face-to-face assessment.

By implementing the principles in this book, we can facilitate the client to be as independent as they can be and the care worker to go home injury free. As allied health professionals, we can feel confident in the advice we have provided.

The HoistEd Program

HOIST ED

Are you ready to join the thousands of health professionals who are helping keep care workers injury free?

HoistEd is a 12-week program designed for allied health professionals to learn the knowledge, skills and resources in manual handling to keep care workers injury free.

The program is designed to help you implement the 10 principles covered in this book, link in with other allied health professionals and learn from experts in the field.

Over one thousand allied health professionals around the world have already used this program to enhance their skills in the prevention of injury in the care of people with complex physical disabilities.

For more information on the HoistEd program visit:

www.riskmanaged.com.au/hoisted

Next steps

Several resources are available to support you developing the skill set to keep care workers injury free:

- *Lunch 'n' learns:* These are 1.5-hour sessions we regularly deliver in partnership with equipment companies as a way of offering powerful bite-size messages to start you on your way to enhancing your skills in the prevention of injury in the care of people with disabilities.

- *Webinars:* We offer regular webinars through our website (www.riskmanaged.com.au).

- *HoistEd:* Our flagship 12-week program is ideal for health professionals looking to gain the ultimate knowledge, skills and resources to keep care workers injury free.

To find out more, visit **www.riskmanaged.com.au**

Notes

Notes

Notes

Notes

Notes

Notes